THOMSON DELMAR LEARNING'S NURSING REVIEW SERIES

Psychiatric Nursing

Content taken from:
NCLEX-RN® Review

By:
Alice M. Stein EdD, RN
Retired
Senior Associate Dean for Student and Business Affairs
Drexel University
College of Nursing and Health Professions
Philadelphia, Pennsylvania

THOMSON

DELMAR LEARNING Australia Canada Mexico Singapore Spain United Kingdom United States

THOMSON

™

DELMAR LEARNING

Nursing Review Series: Psychiatric Nursing

by Alice M. Stein

Vice President, Health Care Business Unit:
William Brottmiller

Director of Learning Solutions:
Matthew Kane

Acquisitions Editor:
Tamara Caruso

Product Manager:
Patricia Gaworecki

Editorial Assistant:
Jenn Waters

Marketing Director:
Jennifer McAvey

Marketing Channel Manager:
Michele McTighe

Marketing Coordinator:
Danielle Pacella

Technology Director:
Laurie Davis

Technology Project Manager:
Mary Colleen Liburdi
Patricia Allen

Production Director:
Carolyn Miller

Production Manager:
Barbara Bullock

Art Director:
Robert Plante
Jack Pendleton

Content Project Manager:
Dave Buddle
Stacey Lamodi
Jessica McNavich

Production Coordinator:
Mary Ellen Cox

COPYRIGHT © 2007
Thomson Delmar Learning,
a part of the Thomson
Corporation. Thomson, the Star
logo, and Delmar Learning are
trademarks used herein under
license.

Printed in the United States
1 2 3 4 5 6 7 8 XXX 09 08 07 06 05

For more information, contact
Thomson Delmar Learning,
5 Maxwell Drive,
Clifton Park, NY 12065
Or find us on the World Wide
Web at
http://www.delmarlearning.com

Library of Congress Cataloging-
in-Publication Data
ISBN 1-4018-1178-7

Contents

Appendices

Contributors

Margaret Ahearn-Spera, RN, C, MSN
Director, Medical Patient Care Services
Danbury Hospital
Danbury, Connecticut
Assistant Clinical Professor
Yale University School of Nursing
New Haven, Connecticut

Mary Mescher Benbenek, RN, MS, CPNP, CFNP
Teaching Specialist
School of Nursing
University of Minnesota
Twin Cities, Minnesota

Cynthia Blank-Reid, RN, MSN, CEN
Trauma Clinical Nurse Specialist
Temple University Hospital
Philadelphia, Pennsylvania
Clinical Adjunct Associate Professor
Drexel University College of Nursing and
    Health Professions
Philadelphia, Pennsylvania

Elizabeth Blunt, PhD (c), MSN
Assistant Professor and Director,
    Graduate Nursing Programs
Drexel University College of Nursing and
    Health Professions
Philadelphia, Pennsylvania

Margaret Brenner, RN, MSN
Senior Consultant, Pinnacle Healthcare
    Group, Inc.
Paoli, Pennsylvania

Margaret Brogan, RN, BSN
Registered Nurse/Expert
Children's Memorial Hospital
Chicago, Illinois

Mary Lynn Burnett, RN, PhD
Assistant Professor of Nursing
Wichita State University
Wichita, Kansas

Corine K. Carlson, RN, MS
Assistant Professor
Department of Nursing
Luther College
Decorah, Iowa

Nancy Clarkson, MEd, RN, BC
Professor and Chairperson
Department of Nursing
Finger Lakes Community College
Canandaigua, New York

Nancy Clarkson, RN, C, MEd
Associate Professor of Nursing
Finger Lakes Community College
Canandaigua, New York

Gretchen Reising Cornell, RN, PhD, CNE
Professor of Nursing
Utah Valley State College
Orem, Utah

Vera V. Cull, RN, DSN
Former Assistant Professor of Nursing
University of Alabama
Birmingham, Alabama

Deborah L. Dalrymple, RN, MSN, CRNI
Associate Professor of Nursing
Montgomery County Community College
Blue Bell, Pennsylvania

Laura DeHelian, RN, PhD, APRN, BC
Former Assistant Professor of Nursing
Cleveland State University
Cleveland, Ohio

Della J. Derscheid, RN, MS, CNS
Assistant Professor
Department of Nursing
Mayo Clinic
Mayo Clinic College of Nursing
Rochester, Minnesota

Judy Donlen, RN, DNSc
Executive Director, Southern New Jersey
Perinatal Cooperative
Pennsauken, New Jersey

Judith L. Draper, APRN, BC
Assistant Professor
Drexel University College of Nursing and
    Health Professions
Philadelphia, Pennsylvania

Theresa M. Fay-Hillier, MSN, RN, CS
Adjunct Faculty
Drexel University College of Nursing and
    Health Professions
Philadelphia, Pennsylvania

Marcia R. Gardner, MA, RN, CPNP, CPN
Assistant Professor
Drexel University College of Nursing and
    Health Professions
Philadelphia, Pennsylvania

Ann Garey, MSN, APRN, BC, FNP
Carle Foundation Hospital
Urbana, Illinois

Jeanne Gelman, RN, MA, MSN
Professor Emeritus, Psychiatric-Mental
    Health Nursing
Widener University
Chester, Pennsylvania

Theresa M. Giglio, RD, MS
Instructor, LaSalle University
Philadelphia, Pennsylvania

Beth Good, RN, MSN, BSN
Teaching Specialist
University of Minnesota
Minneapolis, Minnesota

Samantha Grover, RN, BSN, CNS
Psychiatric Mental Health Clinical
    Specialist
MeritCare Health System
Moorhead, Minnesota

Judith M. Hall, RNC, MSN, IBCLC, LCCE
Lactation Consultant and Childbirth
    Educator
Mary Washington Hospital
Fredericksburg, Virginia

**Judith M. Hall, RNC, MSN, IBCLC,
LCCE, FACCE**
Mary Washington Hospital
Fredericksburg, Virginia

**Jeanne M. Harkness, RN, BA, MSN,
BSN, AOCN**
Clinical Practice Specialist
Jane Brattain Breast Center
Park Nicollet Clinic
St. Louis Park, Minnesota

Marilyn Herbert-Ashton, RN, C, MS
Director, Wellness Center
F. F. Thompson Health Systems, Inc.
Adjunct Professor of Nursing
Finger Lakes Community College
Canandaigua, New York

Marilyn Herbert-Ashton, MS, RN, BC
Virginia Western Community College
Roanoke, VA

Holly Hillman, RN, MSN
Assistant Professor
Montgomery County Community College
Blue Bell, Pennsylvania

Lorraine C. Igo, RN, MSN, EdD
Assistant Professor
Drexel University College of Nursing and
    Health Professions
Philadelphia, Pennsylvania

Linda Irle, RN, MSN, APN, CNP
Coordinator, Maternal-Child Nursing
University of Illinois
Urbana, Illinois
Family Nurse Practitioner, Acute Care,
Carle Clinic,
Champaign, Illinois

Amy Jacobson, RN, BA
Staff Nurse
United Hospital
St. Paul, Minnesota

Nancy H. Jacobson, MSN, APRN-BC, CS
Staff Development Coordinator
Rydal Park
Rydal, Pennsylvania

Nancy H. Jacobson, RN, CS, MSN
Senior Manager
The Whitman Group
Huntington Valley, Pennsylvania

Nadine James, RN, PhD
Assistant Professor of Nursing
University of Southern Mississippi
Hattiesburg, Mississippi

Lisa Jensen, CS, MS, APRN
Salt Lake City VA Healthcare System
Salt Lake City, Utah

Ellen Joswiak, RN, MA
Assistant Professor of Nursing
Staff Nurse
Mayo Medical Center
Rochester, Minnesota

Charlotte D. Kain, RN, C, EdD
Professor Nursing, Health Care of Women
Montgomery County Community College
Blue Bell, Pennsylvania

Roseann Tirotta Kaplan, MSN, RN, CS
Adjunct Faculty
Drexel University College of Nursing and
    Health Professions
Philadelphia, Pennsylvania

Betsy Ann Skrha Kennedy, RN, MS, CS, LCCE
Nursing Instructor
Rochester Community and Technical
    College
Rochester, Minnesota

Robin M. Lally, PhD, RN, BA, AOCN, CNS
Teaching Specialist; Office 6-155
School of Nursing
University of Minnesota
Twin Cities, Minnesota

Penny Leake, RN, PhD
Luther College
Decorah, Iowa

Barbara Mandleco, RN, PhD
Associate Professor & Undergraduate
    Program Coordinator
College of Nursing
Brigham Young University
Provo, Utah

Mary Lou Manning, RN, PhD, CPNP
Director, Infection Control and
    Occupational Health
The Children's Hospital of Philadelphia
Adjunct Assistant Professor
University of Pennsylvania School of
    Nursing
Philadelphia, Pennsylvania

Gerry Matsumura, RN, PhD, MSN, BSN
Former Associate Professor of Nursing
Brigham Young University
Provo, Utah

Alberta McCaleb, RN, DSN
Associate Professor
Chair, Undergraduate Studies
University of Alabama School of Nursing
University of Alabama at Birmingham
Birmingham, Alabama

Judith C. Miller, RN, MSN
President, Nursing Tutorial and
    Consulting Services
Clifton, Virginia

Eileen Moran, RN, C, MSN
Clinical Educator
Abington Memorial Hospital
Abington, Pennsylvania

JoAnn Mulready-Shick, RN, MS
Dean, Nursing and Allied Health
Roxbury Community College
Boston, Massachusetts

Patricia Murdoch, RN, MS
Nurse Practitioner
University of Illinois, Chicago
Urbana, Illinois

Jayme S. Nelson, RN, MS, ARNP-C
Adult Nurse Practitioner
Assistant Professor of Nursing
Luther College
Decorah, Iowa

Janice Nuuhiwa, MSN, CPON, APN/CNS
Staff Development Specialist
Hematology/Oncology/Stem Cell
    Transplant Division
Children's Memorial Hospital
Chicago, Illinois

Kristen L. Osborn, MSN, CRNP
Pediatric Nurse Specialist
UAB School of Nursing
UAB Pediatric Hematology/Oncology
Birmingham, Alabama

Marie O'Toole, RN, EdD
Associate Professor, College of Nursing
Rutgers, The State University of New Jersey
Newark, New Jersey

Faye A. Pearlman, RN, MSN, MBA
Assistant Professor
Drexel University College of Nursing and
    Health Professions
Philadelphia, Pennsylvania

Karen D. Peterson, RN, MSN, BSN, PNP
Pediatric Nurse Practitioner
Division of Endocrinology
Children's Memorial Hospital
Chicago, Illinois

Kristin Sandau, RN, PhD
Bethel University's Department of
    Nursing
United's John Nasseff Heart Hospital
Minneapolis, Minnesota

Elizabeth Sawyer, RN, BSN, CCRN
Registered Nurse
United Hospital
St. Paul, Minnesota

Lisa A. Seldomridge, RN, PhD
Associate Professor of Nursing
Salisbury University
Salisbury, Maryland

Janice Selekman, RN, DNSc
Professor and Chair
Department of Nursing
University of Delaware
Newark, Delaware

Robert Shearer, CRNA, MSN
Assistant Professor
Drexel University College of Nursing and
    Health Professions
Philadelphia, Pennsylvania

Constance O. Kolva Taylor, RN, MSN
Kolva Consulting
Harrisburg, Pennsylvania

Magdeleine Vasso, MSN, RN
Assistant Professor
Drexel University College of Nursing and
    Health Professions
Philadelphia, Pennsylvania

Janice L. Vincent, RN, DSN
University of Alabama School of Nursing
University of Alabama at Birmingham
Birmingham, Alabama

Margaret Vogel, RN, MSN, BSN
Nursing Instructor
Rochester Community & Technical
    College
Rochester, Minnesota

Anne Robin Waldman, RN, C, MSN, AOCN
Clinical Nurse Specialist
Albert Einstein Medical Center
Philadelphia, Pennsylvania

Mary Shannon Ward, RN, MSN
Children's Memorial Hospital
Chicago, Illinois

Virginia R. Wilson, RN, MSN, CEN
Assistant Professor, Graduate Nursing
    Programs
Drexel University College of Nursing and
    Health Professions
Philadelphia, Pennsylvania

Preface

Congratulations on discovering the best new review series for the NCLEX-RN®! Thomson Delmar Learning's Nursing Review Series is designed to maximize your study in the core subject areas covered on the NCLEX-RN® examination. The series consists of 8 books:

Pharmacology

Medical-Surgical Nursing

Pediatric Nursing

Maternity and Women's Health Nursing

Gerontologic Nursing

Psychiatric Nursing

Legal and Ethical Nursing

Community Health Nursing

Each text has been developed expressly to meet your needs as you study and prepare for the all-important licensure examination. Taking this exam is a stressful event and constitutes a major career milestone. Passing the NCLEX is the key to your future ability to practice as a registered nurse.

Each text in the series is designed around the most current test plan for the NCLEX-RN® and provides a focused and complete content review in each subject area. Additionally, there are up to 400 review questions in each text: questions at the end of most every chapter and three 100 question review tests that support the chapter content. Each set of review questions is followed by answers and rationales for both the right and wrong answers. There is also a free PDA download of review questions available with the purchase of any of these review texts! It is this combination of content review and self assessment that provides a powerful learning experience for you as you prepare for you examination.

ORGANIZATION

Thomson Delmar Learning's unique Pharmacology review book provides you with an intensive review in this all important subject area. Drugs are grouped by classification and similarities to aid you in consolidating this pertinent but sometimes overwhelming information. Included in this text are:

- A section on herbal medicines, now being tested on the exam.
- Case studies that apply relevant drug content
- Prototypes for most drug classifications
- Mechanism of drug action
- Uses and adverse effects
- Nursing implications and discharge teaching
- Related drugs and their variance from the prototype

The review texts for Medical-Surgical Nursing, Pediatric Nursing, Maternity Nursing, Gerontological Nursing and Psychiatric Nursing follow a systematic approach that includes:

- The nursing process integrated with a body systems approach
- Introductory review of normal anatomy and physiology as well as basic theories and principles
- Review of pertinent disorders for each system including: general characteristics, pathophysiology/psychopathology
- Medical management
- Assessment data
- Nursing interventions and client education

Community Health Nursing and Legal and Ethical Nursing are unique review texts in the marketplace. They include aspects of community health nursing and legal/ethical subject matter that is covered on the NCLEX-RN® exam. Community Health topics covered are: case management, long-term care, home health care and hospice. Legal and ethical topics include: cultural diversity, leadership and management, ethical issues and legal issues for older adults.

FEATURES

All questions in each text in the series are compliant with the most current test plan from the National Council of State Boards of Nursing (NCSBN). All questions are followed by answers and rationales for both right and wrong choices. Included are many of the alternative format questions first introduced to the exam in 2003. An icon identifies these alternate types ⊙. The questions in each of these texts are written primarily at the application or analysis cognitive levels allowing you to further enhance critical thinking skills which are heavily weighted on the NCLEX.

In addition, with the purchase of any of these texts, a free PDA download is available to you. It provides you with up to an additional 225 questions with which you can practice your test taking skills.

Thomson Delmar Learning is committed to help you reach your fullest professional potential. Good luck on the NCLEX-RN® examination!

To access your free PDA download for Thomson Delmar Learning's Nursing Review Series visit the online companion resource at **www.delmarhealthcare.com** Click on Online Companions then select the Nursing discipline.

Reviewers

Judy Bourrand, RN, MSN
Ida V. Moffett School of Nursing
Samford University
Birmingham, Alabama

Mary Kathie Doyle, BS, CCRN,
Instructor
Maria College
Troy, New York

Mary Lashley, PhD, RN, CS
Associate Professor
Towson University
Towson, Maryland

Melissa Lickteig, EdD, RN
Instructor, School of Nursing
Georgia Southern University
Statesboro, Georgia

Darlene Mathis, MSN, RN APRN, BC,
NP-C, CRNP
Assistant Professor
Ida V. Moffett School of Nursing
Samford University
Birmingham, Alabama

Barbara McGraw, MSN, RN
Instructor
Central Community College
Grand Island, Nebraska

Carol Meadows, MNSc, RNP, APN
Eleanor Mann School of Nursing
University of Arkansas
Fayetteville, Arkansas

Maria Smith, DSN, RN, CCRN
Professor, School of Nursing
Middle Tennessee State University
Murfreesboro, Tennessee

1

Overview of Psychiatric-Mental Health Nursing

■ THEORETICAL BASIS

Medical-Biologic Model

A. Emotional distress is viewed as illness.
B. Symptoms can be classified to determine a psychiatric diagnosis.
C. DSM IV-TR*
   1. Description of disorders
   2. Criteria (behaviors) that must be met for diagnosis to be made
   3. Axis: the dimensions and factors included when assessing a client with a mental disorder
      a. I and II: clinical syndromes (e.g., bipolar, antisocial personality, mental retardation)
      b. III: physical disorders and symptoms (e.g., cystic fibrosis, hypertension)
      c. IV: psychosocial and environmental problems: acute and long-term severity of stressors
      d. V: functioning of client, rating of symptoms and their effect on activities of daily living (ADL) or violence to self/others
D. Diagnosed psychiatric illnesses are within the realm of medical practice and have a particular course, prognosis, and treatment regimen.
E. Treatment can include psychotropic drugs, electroconvulsive therapy (ECT), hospitalization, and psychotherapy.
F. There is no proven cause, but theory is that biochemical/genetic factors play a part in the development of mental illness. Theories with schizophrenia and affective disorders include
   1. Genetic: increased risk when close relative (e.g., parent, sibling) has disorder
   2. Possible link to neurotransmitter activity

*American Psychiatric Association. (2000). *Diagnostic and Statistical Manual of Mental Disorders* (4th ed.), Text Revision.

Psychodynamic/Psychoanalytic Model (Freud)

A. Instincts (drives) produce energy.
B. There are genetically determined drives for sex and aggression.
C. Human behavior is determined by past experiences and responses.
D. All behavior has meaning and can be understood.
E. Emotionally painful experiences/anxiety motivate behavior.
F. Client can change behavior and responses when made aware of the reasons for them.
G. Freud's theory of personality
   1. *Id*: present at birth; instinctual drive for pleasure and immediate gratification, unconscious. *Libido* is the sexual and/or aggressive energy (drive). Operates on pleasure principle to reduce tension or discomfort (pain). Uses *primary process* thinking by imagining objects to satisfy needs (hallucinating).
   2. *Ego*: develops as sense of self that is distinct from world of reality; conscious, preconscious, and unconscious. Operates on reality principle which determines whether the perception has a basis in reality or is imagined. Uses *secondary* process thinking by judging reality and solving problems.
      a. Functions of the ego
         1) control and regulate instinctual drives
         2) mediate between id drives and demands of reality; id drives vs superego restrictions
         3) reality testing: evaluate and judge external world
         4) store up experiences in "memory"
         5) direct motor activity and actions
         6) solve problems
         7) use defense mechanisms to protect self
      b. Levels of awareness
         1) Preconscious: knowledge not readily available to conscious awareness but can be brought to awareness with effort (e.g., recalling name of a character in a book)
         2) Unconscious: knowledge that cannot be brought into conscious awareness without interventions such as psychoanalysis, hypnotism, or drugs
         3) Conscious: aware of own thoughts and perceptions of reality
   3. *Superego*: develops as person unconsciously incorporates standards and restrictions from parents to guide behaviors, thoughts, and feelings. Conscious awareness of acceptable/unacceptable thoughts, feelings, and actions is "conscience."
H. Freud's psychosexual developmental stages
   1. *Oral*
      a. 0-18 months
      b. Pleasure and gratification through mouth

      c. Behaviors: dependency, eating, crying, biting

      d. Distinguishes between self and mother

      e. Develops body image, aggressive drives

  2. *Anal*

      a. 18 months–3 years

      b. Pleasure through elimination or retention of feces

      c. Behaviors: control of holding on or letting go

      d. Develops concept of power, punishment, ambivalence, concern with cleanliness or being dirty

  3. *Phallic/Oedipal*

      a. 3-6 years

      b. Pleasure through genitals

      c. Behaviors: touching of genitals, erotic attachment to parent of opposite sex

      d. Develops fear of punishment by parent of same sex, guilt, sexual identity

  4. *Latency*

      a. 6-12 years

      b. Energy used to gain new skills in social relationships and knowledge

      c. Behaviors: sense of industry and mastery

      d. Learns control over aggressive, destructive impulses

      e. Acquires friends

  5. *Genital*

      a. 12-20 years

      b. Sexual pleasure through genitals

      c. Behaviors: becomes independent of parents, responsible for self

      d. Develops sexual identity, ability to love and work

Psychosocial Model (Erikson)

A. Emphasis on psychosocial rather than psychosexual development

B. Developmental stages have goals (tasks)

C. Challenge in each stage is to resolve conflict (e.g., trust vs mistrust)

D. Resolution of conflict prepares individual for next developmental stage

E. Personality develops according to biologic, psychologic, and social influences

F. Erikson's psychosocial development tasks

  1. *Trust vs mistrust*

      a. 0-18 months

      b. Learn to trust others and self vs withdrawal, estrangement

  2. *Autonomy vs shame and doubt*

      a. 18 months–3 years

      b. Learn self-control and the degree to which one has control over the environment vs compulsive compliance or defiance

3. *Initiative vs guilt*
   a. 3–5 years
   b. Learn to influence environment, evaluate own behavior vs fear of doing wrong, lack of self-confidence, overrestricting actions
4. *Industry vs inferiority*
   a. 6–12 years
   b. Creative; develop sense of competency vs sense of inadequacy
5. *Identity vs role diffusion*
   a. 12–20 years
   b. Develop sense of self; preparation, planning for adult roles vs doubts relating to sexual identity, occupation/career
6. *Intimacy vs isolation*
   a. 18–25 years
   b. Develop intimate relationship with another; commitment to career vs avoidance of choices in relationships, work, or lifestyle
7. *Generativity vs stagnation*
   a. 21–45 years
   b. Productive; use of energies to guide next generation vs lack of interests, concern with own needs
8. *Integrity vs despair*
   a. 45 years to end of life
   b. Relationships extended, belief that own life has been worthwhile vs lack of meaning of one's life, fear of death

Interpersonal Model (Sullivan)

A. Behavior motivated by need to avoid anxiety and satisfy needs
B. Sullivan's developmental tasks
   1. *Infancy*
      a. 0–18 months
      b. Others will satisfy needs
   2. *Childhood*
      a. 18 months–6 years
      b. Learn to delay need gratification
   3. *Juvenile*
      a. 6–9 years
      b. Learn to relate to peers
   4. *Preadolescence*
      a. 9–12 years
      b. Learn to relate to friends of same sex
   5. *Early adolescence*
      a. 12–14 years
      b. Learn independence and how to relate to opposite sex
   6. *Late adolescence*
      a. 14–21 years
      b. Develop intimate relationship with person of opposite sex

Therapeutic Nurse-Client Relationship (Peplau)

A. Based on Sullivan's interpersonal model

B. Therapeutic relationship is between nurse (helper) and client (recipient of care). The goal is to work together to assist client to grow and to resolve problems.

C. Differs from social relationship where both parties form alliance for mutual benefit.

D. Therapeutic use of self

    1. Focus is on client needs but nurse is also aware of own needs.

    2. Self-awareness enables nurse to avoid having own needs influence perception of client.

    3. Determine what client/family needs are at the time.

E. Three phases of nurse-client relationship

    1. *Orientation*

        a. Nurse explains relationship to client, defines both nurse's and client's roles.

        b. Nurse determines what client expects from the relationship and what can be done for the client.

        c. Nurse contracts with client about when and where future meetings will take place.

        d. Nurse assesses client and develops a plan of care based on appropriate nursing diagnoses.

        e. Limits/termination of relationship are introduced (e.g., "We will be meeting for 30 minutes every morning while you are in the hospital.").

    2. *Working phase*

        a. Client's problems and needs are identified and explored as nurse and client develop mutual acceptance.

        b. Client's dysfunctional symptoms, feelings, or interpersonal relationships are identified.

        c. Therapeutic techniques are employed to reduce anxiety and to promote positive change and independence.

        d. Goals are evaluated as therapeutic work proceeds, and changed as determined by client's progress.

    3. *Termination*

        a. Relationship and growth in nurse and client are summarized.

        b. Client may become anxious and react with increased dependence, hostility, or withdrawal.

        c. These reactions are discussed with client.

        d. Feelings of nurse and client concerning termination should be discussed in context of finiteness of relationship.

F. Transference and countertransference

    1. *Transference*: occurs when client transfers conflicts/feelings from past to the nurse. *Example:* Client becomes overly dependent, clinging to nurse who represents (unconsciously to client) the nurturing client desires from own mother.

2. *Countertransference*: occurs when nurse responds to client emotionally, as if in a personal, not professional/therapeutic, relationship. Countertransference is a normal occurrence, but must be recognized so that supervision or consultation can keep it from undermining the nurse-client relationship. *Example:* Nurse is sarcastic and judgmental to client who has history of drug abuse. Client represents (unconsciously to nurse) the nurse's brother who has abused drugs.
3. Interventions
    a. Reflect on reasons for behaviors of client or nurse.
    b. Establish therapeutic goals for this relationship.
    c. If unable to control these occurrences, transfer client to another nurse.

Human Motivation/Need Model (Maslow)

A. Hierarchy of needs in order of importance
    1. Physiologic: oxygen, food, water, sleep, sex
    2. Safety: security, protection, freedom from anxiety
    3. Love and belonging: freedom from loneliness/alienation
    4. Esteem and recognition: freedom from sense of worthlessness, inferiority, and helplessness
    5. Self-actualization: aesthetic needs, self-fulfillment, creativity, spirituality
B. Primary needs (oxygen, fluids) need to be met prior to dealing with higher-level needs (esteem, recognition).
C. Focus on provision of positive aspects such as feeling safe, having someone care, affiliation

Behavioral Model (Pavlov, Skinner)

A. Behavior is learned and retained by positive reinforcement.
B. Motivation for behavior is not considered.
C. Behaviors that are not adequate can be replaced by more adaptive behaviors.

Community Mental Health Model

A. Emotional distress stems from personal and social factors
    1. Family problems (e.g., divorce, single parenthood)
    2. Social factors (e.g., unemployment, lack of support groups, changing mores)
B. Health care a right
C. Decreased need for hospitalization, increased community care
D. Collaboration of social and health care services
E. Comprehensive services
    1. Emergency care
    2. Inpatient/outpatient services

3. Substance-abuse treatment
4. Transitional living arrangements (temporary residence instead of inpatient care)
5. Consultation and education to increase knowledge of mental health
F. Prevention
1. Primary prevention
   a. Minimize development of serious emotional distress: promote mental health, identify persons at risk.
   b. Anticipate problems such as developmental crises (e.g., birth of first child, midlife crisis, death of spouse).
2. Secondary prevention: early case finding and treatment (drug therapy, outpatient, short-term hospitalization).
3. Tertiary prevention: restore client to optimal functioning; facilitate return of client to home and community by use of social agencies.

■ NURSING PROCESS

A. Applies to all clients, not only to those with psychiatric diagnosis; incorporates holism.
B. Utilized in a unique manner for psychosocial assessment.
C. Sets goals (with client, whenever possible) that can be measured in behavioral terms (e.g., client will dress self and eat breakfast before 9 A.M.).
D. Uses principles of therapeutic communication for interventions.
E. Evaluates whether, how well goals were met.

Physical Assessment

A. Subjective reporting of health history
B. Objective data (general status and appearance)
1. Age: client's appearance in relation to chronologic age
2. Attire: appropriateness of clothing to age/ situation
3. Hygiene: cleanliness and grooming, or lack thereof
4. Physical health: weight, physical distress
5. Psychomotor: posture, movement, activity level
6. Sleep and rest
C. Neurologic assessment/level of consciousness

Mental Status Assessment

Emotional Status Assessment

Observation of mood (prolonged emotion) and affect (physical manifestations of mood). That is, sad mood may be evidenced by crying or downcast appearance; joyful mood may be expressed by smiling or happy affect.

A. Appropriateness
B. Description: flat, sad, smiling, serious
C. Stability
D. Specific feelings and moods

Cognitive Assessment

Evaluation of thought, sensorium, intelligence

A. Intellectual performance
    1. Orientation to person, place, and time
    2. Attention and concentration
    3. Knowledge/educational level
    4. Memory: short and long term
    5. Judgment
    6. Insight into illness
    7. Ability to use abstraction
B. Speech
    1. Amount, volume, clarity
    2. Characteristics: pressured, slow or fast, dull or lively
    3. Specific aberrations, i.e., echolalia (imitating and repeating another's words or phrases) or neologisms (making up of own words that have special meaning to client).
C. Thoughts
    1. Content and clarity
    2. Characteristics: spontaneity, speed, loose associations, blocked, flight of ideas, repetitions

Social/Cultural Considerations

A. Age: assess for developmental tasks and developmental crises, age-related problems.
    1. 0–18 months: development of trust and sense of self, dependency
    2. 18 months–3 years: development of autonomy and beginning self-reliance, toilet training
    3. 3–6 years: development of sexual identity, relationships with peers, adjustment to school
    4. 6–12 years: mastery of skills, beginning self-esteem, identification with others outside family, social relationships
    5. 12–18 years: sense of self solidifies, separation and individuation often follow some disorganization and rebellion, substance abuse
    6. 18–25 years: identification with peer group, setting of personal and career goals to master future
    7. 25–38 years: take place in adult world, commitments made relating to career, marriage, parenthood
    8. 38–65 years: review of past accomplishments; may set new and reasonable goals; midlife crises when present achievements have not met goals set in earlier stages of development
    9. 65/70 to death: loss of friends/spouse, retirement, loss of some social/physical functions
B. Family/community relationships
    1. Role of client in family
    2. Family harmony, family support for or dependency on client

3. Client's perception of family
4. Availability of community support groups to client (include government social agencies; religious, ethnic, and volunteer agencies)

C. Socioeconomic group/education
1. Factors that relate to how client is approached and how client perceives own present state
2. Determination of level of teaching and need for social services

D. Cultural/spiritual background
1. Assess behaviors in context of client's culture.
2. Avoid stereotyping persons as having attributes of their culture/ subculture.
3. Note client's religious/philosophic beliefs.

■ ANALYSIS

Select nursing diagnoses based on collected data. Decide which is most important. Specific nursing diagnoses will be given when discussing particular disorders, but those nursing diagnoses generally appropriate to the client with psychiatric-mental health disorders include

A. Anxiety
B. Ineffective coping
C. Decisional conflict
D. Fatigue
E. Fear
F. Hopelessness
G. Deficient knowledge
H. Powerlessness
I. Disturbed sleep pattern
J. Disturbed thought processes
K. Risk for violence
L. Impaired verbal communication
M. Impaired social interaction
N. Ineffective role performance
O. Spiritual distress
P. Low self-esteem
Q. Social isolation
R. Dysfunctional family processes
S. Defensive coping
T. Ineffective denial
U. Noncompliance
V. Disturbed body image
W. Risk for injury
X. Rape-trauma syndrome
Y. Impaired adjustment

■ PLANNING AND IMPLEMENTATION

Goals

A. Client will
  1. Participate in treatment program.
  2. Be oriented to time, place, and person and exhibit reality-based behavior.
  3. Recognize reasons for behavior and develop alternative coping mechanisms.
  4. Maintain or improve self-care activities.
  5. Be protected from harmful behaviors.
B. There will be mutual agreement of nurse and client whenever possible.
C. Short-term goals are set for immediate problems; they should be feasible and within client's capabilities.
D. Long-term goals are related to discharge planning and prevention of recurrence or exacerbation of symptoms.

Interventions

The nurse will use therapeutic intervention and the nurse-client relationship to help the client achieve the goals of therapy. Interventions must be geared to the level of the client's capability and must relate to the specific problems identified for the individual client, family, or group.

Therapeutic Communication

A. Facilitative: use the following approaches to intervene therapeutically
  1. Silence: client able to think about self/problems; does not feel pressure or obligation to speak.
  2. Offering self: offer to provide comfort to client by presence (*Nurse:* "I'll sit with you." "I'll walk with you.").
  3. Accepting: indicate nonjudgmental acceptance of client and his perceptions by nodding and following what client says.
  4. Giving recognition: indicate to client your awareness of him and his behaviors (*Nurse:* "Good morning, John. You have combed your hair this morning.").
  5. Making observations: verbalize what you perceive (*Nurse:* "I notice that you can't seem to sit still.").
  6. Encouraging description: ask client to verbalize his perception (*Nurse:* "Tell me when you need to get up and walk around." "What is happening to you now?").
  7. Using broad openings: encourage client to introduce topic of conversation (*Nurse:* "Where shall we begin today?" "What are you thinking about?").

8. Offering general leads: encourage client to continue discussing topic (*Nurse:* "And then?" "Tell me more about that.").
9. Reflecting: direct client's questions/ statements back to encourage expression of ideas and feelings (*Client:* "Do you think I should call my father?" *Nurse:* "What do you want to do?").
10. Restating: repeat what client has said (*Client:* "I don't want to take the medicine." *Nurse:* "You don't want to take this medication?").
11. Focusing: encourage client to stay on topic/point (*Nurse:* "You were talking about . . .").
12. Exploring: encourage client to express feelings or ideas in more depth (*Nurse:* "Tell me more about . . ." "How did you respond to . . . ?").
13. Clarification: encourage client to make idea or feeling more explicit, understandable (*Nurse:* "I don't understand what you mean. Could you explain it to me?").
14. Presenting reality: report events/situations as they really are (*Client:* "I don't get to talk to my doctor." *Nurse:* "I saw your doctor talking to you this morning.").
15. Translating into feelings: encourage client to verbalize feelings expressed in another way (*Client:* "I will never get better." *Nurse:* "You sound rather hopeless and helpless.").
16. Suggesting collaboration: offer to work with client toward goal (*Client:* "I fail at everything I try." *Nurse:* "Maybe we can figure out something together so that you can accomplish something you want to do.").

B. Ineffective communication styles: the following nontherapeutic approaches tend to block therapeutic communication and are sometimes used by nurses to avoid becoming involved with client's emotional distress; often a protective action on part of nurse.
1. Reassuring: telling client there is no need to worry or be anxious (*Client:* "I'm nervous about this test." *Nurse:* "Everything will be all right.").
2. Advising: telling client what you believe should be done (*Client:* "I am going to . . ." *Nurse:* "Why don't you do . . . instead?" or "I think you should do . . .").
3. Requesting explanation: asking client to provide reasons for his feelings/behavior. The use of "why" questions should be avoided (*Nurse:* "Why do you feel, think, or act this way?").
4. Stereotypical response: replying to client with meaningless clichés (*Client:* "I hate being in the hospital." *Nurse:* "There's good and bad about everything.").
5. Belittling feelings: minimizing or making light of client's distress or discomfort (*Client:* "I'm so depressed about . . ." *Nurse:* "Everyone feels sad at times.").

6. Defending: protecting person or institutions (*Client:* "Ms. Jones is a rotten nurse." *Nurse:* "Ms. Jones is one of our best nurses.").

7. Approving: giving approval to client's behavior or opinion (*Client:* "I'm going to change my attitude." *Nurse:* "That's good.").

8. Disapproving: telling client certain behavior or opinions do not meet your approval (*Client:* "I am going to sign myself out of here." *Nurse:* "I'd rather you wouldn't do that.").

9. Agreeing: letting client know that you think, feel alike; nurse verbalizes agreement.

10. Disagreeing: letting client know that you do not agree; telling client that you do not believe he is right.

11. Probing: questioning client about a topic he has indicated he does not want to discuss.

12. Denial: refusing to recognize client's perception (*Client:* "I am a hopeless case" *Nurse:* "You are not hopeless. There is always hope.").

13. Changing topic: letting client know you do not want to discuss a problem by introducing a new topic (*Client:* "I am a hopeless case." *Nurse*: "It's time to fill out your menu.").

Therapeutic Groups

A. Groups of clients meet with one or more therapists. They work together to alleviate client problems in
   1. Interpersonal relations/communication
   2. Coping with particular stressors (e.g., ostomy groups)
   3. Self-understanding
B. Purposes
   1. Increase self-awareness
   2. Improve interpersonal relationships
   3. Make changes in behavior
   4. Deal with particular stressors
   5. Enhance teaching/learning
C. Structure of groups
   1. Leader(s) chosen
   2. Selection of members
   3. Size: 5 to 10 members
   4. Physical arrangements
   5. Time/place of meetings
   6. Open: accept members anytime
   7. Closed: do not add new members
D. Group dynamics
   1. System of interactions
   2. Collective activity

TABLE 1-1   Types of Therapeutic Groups

Type	Goal(s)	Example
Task	Accomplish outcome	Select field trip
Teaching/ learning	Gain knowledge/skills	Identify side effects of medications
Social/support	Give and receive support	Postmastectomy clients
Psychotherapy	Insight/behavioral change	Resolve loss
Activity	Increase social interaction/ self-esteem	Grooming, manicures

     3. Process: all activities/interactions
     4. Content: topics discussed
  E. Stages of group development
     1. Beginning stage
        a. Anxiety in new situation
        b. Information given
        c. Group norms established
     2. Middle stage
        a. Group cohesiveness
        b. Members confronting each other
        c. Reliance on group member leading to self-reliance
        d. Sense of trust established
     3. Termination stage
        a. Individual member may leave abruptly
        b. Group decides work is done
        c. Ambivalence felt about termination
        d. Ideally, group members have met goals
  F. Role of the nurse
     1. Explain purpose and rules of group
     2. Introduce group members
     3. Promote group cohesiveness
     4. Focus on problems of group and group process
     5. Encourage participation
     6. Role model
     7. Facilitate communication
     8. Set limits
Table 1-1 lists types of therapeutic groups.

Family Therapy

A. Client is whole family, although a family member may be "identified client."
B. Purposes
  1. Improve relationships among family members
  2. Promote family function
  3. Resolve family problem(s)
C. Process
  1. Problem(s) are identified by each family member.
  2. Members discuss their involvement in problem(s).
  3. Members discuss how problem(s) affect them.
  4. Members explore ways each of them can help resolve problem(s).
D. Role of the nurse
  1. Assess interactions among family members
  2. Make observations to family members
  3. Encourage expression of feelings by family members to one another
  4. Assist family in resolving problems

Milieu Therapy

A. Total environment (milieu) has an effect on individual's behavior, including
  1. Physical environment (i.e., cleanliness, noise, colors, fresh air, light)
  2. Relationships of staff to staff, staff to clients, and client to clients
  3. Atmosphere of safety, caring, mutual respect (e.g., client-run community meeting, community-set standards for behaviors)
B. Purposes
  1. Improve client's behavior
  2. Involve client in decision making of unit
  3. Increase client's sense of autonomy
  4. Increase communication among clients and between clients and staff
  5. Set structure of unit and behavioral limits
  6. Form a sense of community
C. Role of the nurse
  1. Involve clients in decision making
  2. Promote involvement of all staff
  3. Promote development of social skills of individual clients (e.g., nurse serves as role model)
  4. Encourage sense of community in staff and clients

Crisis Intervention

A. Client cannot resolve problem with usual problem-solving skills. Problem is so serious that functioning (homeostasis) is threatened. Crisis can be developmental (e.g., birth of first child), a sudden death (e.g., car accident), a result of interpersonal violence (e.g., arson), terrorist attacks and war (e.g., September 11, 2001), or situational (e.g., home destroyed by fire). Adapting to and coping with the crisis can be considered within the normal range up to 1 year.

B. Purposes
  1. Support client during time of crisis
  2. Resolve crisis
  3. Restore client at least to precrisis level of functioning or assist client to integrate the crisis and reinvest in life
  4. Allow client to attain higher level of functioning through acquiring greater skill in problem solving

C. Process
  1. Crisis event occurs: client unable to solve problem.
  2. Increase in level of client's anxiety.
  3. Client may use trial and error approach.
  4. If problem unresolved, anxiety escalates and client seeks help.

D. Role of the nurse
  1. Assess client's perception of problem: realistic/distorted
  2. Determine situational supports (e.g., family, neighbors, agencies)
  3. Explore previous coping behaviors of client
  4. Offer support and education in resolving crisis
  5. Enlist help of situational supports
  6. Help client develop new, more effective coping behaviors
  7. Convey hope to client that crisis can be resolved
  8. Work with client as he resolves crisis
  9. Encourage the client to attend a debriefing session (if one is available and appropriate for the crisis)

Behavior Modification

A. Based on theory that all behavior is learned as a result of positive reinforcement. Behaviors can be changed by substituting new behaviors.
B. Purpose: change unacceptable or maladaptive behaviors
C. Process
  1. Determine the unacceptable behavior.
  2. Identify more adaptive behavior to replace the unacceptable behavior.
  3. Apply learning principles.
    a. Respond to unacceptable behavior by negative reinforcement (punishment) or by withholding positive reinforcement (ignore behavior).
    b. Determine what client views as reward.
  4. When desired behavior occurs, present positive reinforcement (reward).
  5. Consistently reward desired behavior.
  6. Consistently respond to unacceptable behavior with negative reinforcement/ignoring behavior.

D. Types
  1. *Counterconditioning*: specific stimulus evokes a maladaptive response that is replaced with a more adaptive response.
  2. *Systematic desensitization*
      a. Expose to small amount of stimulus while ensuring relaxation (client cannot be anxious and relaxed at same time).
      b. Continue relaxing client while increasing amount of stimulus.
      c. Fear response to stimulus is eventually extinguished.
  3. *Token economy*: Tokens (rewards such as candy) are used to reinforce desired behaviors.

Psychotropic Medications

A variety of agents is used to control disordered thinking, anxiety, and mood disorders. Effects, side effects, and nursing implications are summarized with each disorder.

■ EVALUATION

A. How well have goals been met? If not met, why not?
  1. Review prior steps of nursing process.
      a. Do you need more assessment data?
      b. Were nursing diagnoses prioritized?
      c. Were goals feasible and measurable?
      d. Were interventions appropriate?
  2. Revise goals as necessary.
B. Client
  1. Enrolled/participates in appropriate treatment program.
  2. Expresses concerns/needs and develops a therapeutic relationship with nurse.
  3. Identifies causes for behavior; learns and uses alternative coping mechanisms.
  4. Demonstrates ability to care for self at optimum level and to identify areas where assistance is needed.
  5. Does not engage in harmful behaviors; shows increased ability to control destructive impulses.
C. Client's behavior demonstrates optimal orientation to reality (e.g., can state name, place); interacts appropriately with others.

■ BEHAVIORS RELATED TO EMOTIONAL DISTRESS

Anxiety

A. General information
  1. One of the most important concepts in psychiatric-mental health nursing.
  2. Anxiety is present in almost every instance where clients are experiencing emotional distress/have a diagnosed psychiatric illness.

NURSING ALERT

Stress can precipitate and increase anxiety.

3. Experienced as a sense of emotional or physical distress as the individual responds to an unknown threat or thwarting of unmet needs.
4. The ego protects itself from the effects of anxiety by the use of defense mechanisms (see Table 1-2).
5. Physiologic responses are related to autonomic nervous system response and to level of anxiety.
   a. Subjective: client experiences feelings of tension, need to act, uneasiness, distress, and apprehension or fear.
   b. Objective: client exhibits restlessness, inability to concentrate, tension, dilated pupils, changes in vital signs (usually increased by sympathetic nervous system response, may be decreased by parasympathetic reactions).
6. Anxiety can be viewed positively (motivates us to change and grow) or negatively (interferes with problem-solving ability and affects functioning).
   a. *Trait anxiety*: individual's normal level of anxiety. Some people are usually rather intense while others are more relaxed; may be related to genetic predisposition/early experiences (repressed conflicts).
   b. *State anxiety*: change in person's anxiety level in response to stressors (environmental or any internal threat to the ego).
7. Levels of anxiety
   a. *Mild*: increased awareness; ability to solve problems, learn; increase in perceptual field; minimal muscle tension
   b. *Moderate*: optimal level for learning, perceptual field narrows to pay attention to particular details, increased tension to solve problems or meet challenges
   c. *Severe*: sympathetic nervous system (flight/fight response); increase in blood pressure, pulse, and respirations; narrowed perceptual field, fixed vision, dilated pupils, can perceive scattered details or only one detail; difficulty in problem solving
   d. *Panic*: decrease in vital signs (release of sympathetic response), distorted perceptual field, inability to solve problems, disorganized behavior, feelings of helplessness/terror
B. Nursing interventions
   1. Determine the level of client's anxiety by assessing verbal and nonverbal behaviors and physiologic symptoms.

TABLE 1-2   Defense Mechanisms

Type	Characteristics	Examples
Denial	Refusal to acknowledge a part of reality	A client on strict bed rest is walking down the hall; shows refusal to acknowledge need to stay in bed because of illness. A client states admission to the mental hospital is for reasons other than mental illness.
Repression	Threatening thoughts are pushed into the unconscious, anxiety and other symptoms are observed; client unable to have conscious awareness of conflicts or events that are source of anxiety	"I don't know why I have to wash my hands all the time, I just have to."
Suppression	Consciously putting a threatening/distressing thought out of one's awareness.	A nurse must study for the NCLEX, but she has had a heated argument with her boyfriend. She decides not to think about the problem until she finishes studying, then she will attempt to resolve it.
Rationalization	Developing an acceptable, justifiable (to self) reason for behavior	A friend tells you that he has been in an automobile accident because the car skidded on wet leaves in the road; you go to the scene of the accident, but there are no leaves; friend admits to you and to self that he was probably driving too fast.
Reaction-formation	Engaging in behavior that is opposite of true desires	A man has an unconscious desire to view pornographic films; he circulates a petition to close the theater where such films are shown.

Sublimation	Anxiety channeled into socially acceptable behavior	A student is upset because she received a failing grade on a test; she knows that she will feel better if she goes jogging and runs a few miles.
Compensation	Making up for a deficit by success in another area	A young man who cannot make any varsity teams becomes the chess champion in his school.
Projection	Placing own undesirable trait onto another; blaming others for own difficulty	A student who would like to cheat on an exam states that other students are trying to cheat; a paranoid client claims that the FBI had him committed to the mental hospital.
Displacement	Directing feelings about one object/person toward a less-threatening object/person	The head nurse reprimands you; you do not argue even though you do not agree with her reprimand; when you return home that evening you are hostile towards your roommate.
Identification	Taking onto oneself the traits of others that one admires	You greatly admire the clinical specialist in your hospital; unconsciously you begin to use the approaches she uses with clients.
Introjection	Symbolic incorporation of another into one's own personality	John becomes depressed when his father dies; John's feelings are directed to the mental image he has of his father.
Conversion	Anxiety converted into a physical symptom that is motor or sensory in nature	A young woman unconsciously desires to strike her mother; she develops sudden paralysis of her arms.

Continued

Table 1-2   Continued

Type	Characteristics	Examples
Symbolization	Representing an idea or object by a substitute object or sign	A man who was spurned by a librarian develops a dislike of books and reading.
Dissociation	Separation or splitting off of one aspect of mental process from conscious awareness	A student who prides herself on being prompt does not recall the times that she arrived late for class.
Undoing	Behavior that is opposite of earlier unacceptable behavior or thought	Joan tells an ethnic joke to a coworker, Sally; Sally, a member of that ethnic group, is offended; the following week Joan offers to work the weekend for Sally.
Regression	Behavior that reflects an earlier level of development; adults hospitalized with serious illnesses sometimes will engage in regressive behaviours	When a new baby is brought home, 5-year-old Billy begins to wet his pants although he had not done this for the past 2½ years.
Isolation	Separating emotional aspects of content from cognitive aspects of thought	A client discusses his terminal diagnosis in clinical terms. He does not express any emotion.
Splitting	Viewing self, others, or situations as all good or all bad	A client tells you that you are the best nurse. Later tells you that you are incompetent and she will report you.

NURSING ALERT

Mild anxiety can serve as a motivator. It can be helpful in serving to increase perception and improves one's ability to see the entire picture.

CLIENT TEACHING CHECKLIST

- Educate the client about their medications, as well as on their administration and safe use.
- Teach progressive relaxation techniques.

2. Determine cause(s) of anxiety with client, if possible.
3. Encourage client to move from affective (feeling) mode to cognitive (thinking) behavior (e.g., ask client, "What are you thinking?"). Stay with client. Reduce anxiety by remaining calm yourself; use silence, or speak slowly and softly.
4. Help client recognize own anxious behavior.
5. Provide outlets (e.g., talking, psychomotor activity, crying, tasks).
6. Provide support and encourage client to find ways to cope with anxiety.
7. In panic state nurse must make decisions.
   a. Do not leave client alone.
   b. Encourage ventilation of thoughts and feelings.
   c. Use firm voice and give short, explicit directions (e.g., "Sit in this chair. I will sit here next to you.").
   d. Engage client in motor activity to reduce tension (e.g., "We can take a brisk walk around the day room. Let's go.").

Defense Mechanisms

Usually unconscious processes used by ego to defend itself from anxiety and threats (see Table 1-2).

Disorders of Perception

Occur with increased anxiety, disordered thinking/impaired reality testing
A. *Illusions*
   1. General information: stimulus in the environment is misperceived (e.g., car backfiring is perceived as a gunshot; a bathrobe in an open closet is perceived as a person in the closet); may be visual, auditory, tactile, gustatory, olfactory.
   2. Nursing intervention: show/explain stimulus to client to promote reality testing.

B. *Delusions*
1. General information: fixed, false set of beliefs that are real to client.
   a. Grandiose: false belief that client has power, wealth, or status or is famous person
   b. Persecutory: false belief that client is the object of another's harassment or harmful intent
   c. Somatic: false belief that client has some physical/physiologic defect
2. Nursing interventions
   a. Avoid arguing: client cannot be convinced, even with evidence, that the belief is false.
   b. Determine client's need (grandiose delusion may indicate low self-esteem; provide opportunities to succeed at task that will enhance self-concept).
   c. Reduce anxiety to encourage decreased need to use delusions.
   d. Accept client's need for delusion, present (but do not insist that client accept) reality.
   e. After therapeutic relationship has been established, you can express doubt about delusions to client.
   f. Direct client's attention to nondelusional, nonthreatening topics (e.g., current events, client's hobbies or interests).

C. *Ideas of reference*
1. General information: belief that events or behaviors of others relate to self (e.g., telephone rings in nurse's station, client believes "they" are calling for him; two nurses are talking and laughing, client believes nurses are talking/laughing at him).
2. Nursing interventions are the same as for delusions.

D. *Hallucinations*
1. General information: sensory perceptions that have no stimulus in environment; most common hallucinations are auditory and visual (e.g., hearing voices; seeing persons, animals, objects).
2. Nursing interventions
   a. Encourage client to describe hallucination.
   b. Accept that this is a real experience for client.
   c. Present reality.
   d. Example: nurse sees client in listening attitude or responding to auditory hallucinations. *Nurse:* "You seem to be listening/talking." *Client:* "The voices are telling me to hurt myself." *Nurse:* "I don't hear the voices. Tell me what the voices are saying to you."

Withdrawal

A. General information: withdrawal from social interaction by not talking, walking away, turning away, sleeping or feigning sleep

B. Nursing interventions
   1. Use silence.
   2. Offer self.
   3. Discuss nonthreatening topics that will not provoke increased anxiety.
   4. Be consistent; keep promises, promote trust.

Hostility and Aggression

A. General information
   1. Hostile behavior: responding to nurse with anger, insults, threats.
   2. Assaultive behavior: attempting to physically harm others.
   3. Usually nurse is not real object of client's anger, but is convenient target for angry feelings/verbalizations.
B. Nursing interventions
   1. Hostility
      a. Recognize own response of anger or defensiveness.
      b. Determine source of client's anger (e.g., intoxicated, psychotic, recent argument with parent).
      c. Accept angry feelings.
      d. Attempt to have client verbalize feelings and channel into acceptable behaviors.
      e. Assess the need for prn medications based on the possible source of the hostility.
   2. Physical aggression/assaultive behaviors (client may act on increased anxiety by throwing objects or attempt to physically harm others)
      a. Assess for increased anxiety.
      b. Maintain distance, at least arm's length.
      c. Attempt to have client verbalize feelings.
      d. Talk client down.
      e. Obtain help if client becomes assaultive.

Self-Mutilation

A. General information: behaviors cause physical injury but are not motivated by the desire to die.
B. Nursing interventions
   1. Assess for suicide risk.
   2. Offer support.
   3. Protect client from carrying out self-mutilation actions.
   4. Remove objects that can be used for self-harm.
   5. Observe for changes in behaviors and attitudes.

Suicide

A. General information
   1. Ideation: verbalization of wish to die (overt or disguised)

TABLE 1-3   Groups at Increased Risk for Suicide

- Adolescents/young adults (ages 15–24)
- Elderly
- Terminally ill
- Persons who have experienced loss/stress
- Survivors of persons who have committed suicide
- Individuals with bipolar disorders
- Depressed persons (when depression begins to lift)
- Substance abusers
- Persons who have attempted suicide previously
- Schizophrenics
- More women attempt suicide; more men complete suicide

2. Gestures: engaging in nonlethal behaviors (e.g., superficial scratches, ingestion of medication in amounts that are not likely to cause serious injury/death)
3. Actions: engaging in behaviors or planning to engage in behaviors that have potential to cause death
4. May or may not be associated with a psychiatric disorder
5. Groups at risk (see Table 1-3)

B. Assessment findings
   1. Verbal cues
      a. Overt: "I'm going to kill myself."
      b. Disguised: "I have the answer to my problems."
   2. Behavioral cues
      a. Giving away prized possessions
      b. Getting financial affairs in order, making a will
      c. Suicidal ideation/gestures
      d. Indications of hopelessness, depression
      e. Behavioral and attitudinal changes (e.g., neat person becomes sloppy, depressed person suddenly becomes alert/positive, increased use of drugs and/or alcohol, alcohol withdrawal).
   3. For lethality assessment, see Table 1-4.

C. Nursing interventions
   1. Contract with client to report suicide ideation with intent and/or suicide attempt.
   2. Assess suicide risk.
      a. Ask client if he thinks about, intends to harm himself.
      b. Ask client if he has formulation of plan; if details are worked out, when? where? how?
      c. Check availability of method (e.g., gun, pills).

TABLE 1-4   Lethality Assessment

- Plans for suicide: when? where? how?
- Means available: what will be used? Is it available to client?
- Lethality of means (e.g., tranquilizers are less lethal when used alone than when combined with alcohol; guns are more lethal than plan to cut wrists)
  - Most lethal: gunshot, hanging, jumping from high places, carbon monoxide, potent poisons (e.g., cyanide)
  - Less lethal: nonprescription drugs, wrist cutting, tranquilizers without CNS depressants
  - Males tend to use more lethal means
- Possibility of "rescue"
- Support systems available or sense of isolation
- Availability of alcohol or drugs
- Severe/panic level of anxiety
- Hostility
- Disorganized thinking
- Preoccupation with thought of suicide plan
- Prior suicide attempts

3. Keep client under constant observation.
4. Remove any objects that can be used in suicide attempt (e.g., shoe laces, sharp objects).
5. Therapeutic intervention
a. Support aspects of wish to live; clients often ambivalent: wish to live and wish to die.
   b. Use one-to-one nurse/client relationship (let client know you care for him).
   c. Allow client to express feelings of hopelessness, helplessness, worthlessness.
   d. Provide hope.
   e. Provide diversionary activities.
   f. Utilize support groups (e.g., family, clergy).
   g. Notify psychiatrist or responsible practitioner for the medical management of the client to evaluate medications and precaution level.
6. Following a suicide
   a. Encourage survivors to discuss client's death, their feelings and fears.
   b. Provide anticipatory guidance to family who may experience problems at holidays, anniversaries.
   c. Hold staff meetings to ventilate feelings and provide a debriefing to process the event.

REVIEW QUESTIONS

1. The nurse is talking with a mother to assess her child. A positive response to which question would indicate the child is in the anal stage of psychosexual development as described by Freud?
   1. "Does he put everything in his mouth?"
   2. "Does he say 'No!' to everything you say?"
   3. "Does he like to dress up and pretend to be his father?"
   4. "Does he seem jealous when you show affection to his father?"

2. The nurse is assessing a 70-year-old woman. Which statement by the client indicates that she has achieved integrity according to Erickson's stages of personality development?
   1. "My life has been wasted."
   2. "My children no longer visit me. I am just waiting to die."
   3. "I was a good nurse when I was younger, but now I am nothing."
   4. "I have a good life and I still enjoy it, but I feel ready to go when it is time."

3. Which cognitive skill would the nurse expect a 6-year-old child to be in the process of developing?
   1. Understanding of basic rules.
   2. Ability to understand abstract concepts.
   3. Recognition of object permanence.
   4. Imitation of others' actions.

4. The nurse is meeting a new client on the unit. Which action, by the nurse, is most effective in initiating the nurse-client relationship?
   1. Introduce self and explain the purpose and the plan for the relationship.
   2. Describe the nurse's family and ask the client to describe his/her family?
   3. Wait until the client indicates a readiness to establish a relationship.
   4. Ask the client why s/he was brought to the hospital.

5. An adult male has just been brought to the psychiatric unit and is pacing up and down the hall. The nurse is to admit him to the hospital. To establish a nurse-client relationship, which approach should the nurse try first?
   1. Assign someone to watch him until he is calmer.
   2. Ask him to sit down and orient him to the nurse's name and the need for information.

3. Check his vital signs, ask him about allergies, and call the physician for sedation.

4. Explain the importance of accurate assessment data to him.

6. The nurse is beginning to establish a nurse-client relationship with a woman who was referred for help in managing her children. The woman arrives late for appointments and focuses on her busy schedule, the difficulty in parking, and other reasons for being late. The nurse best interprets this behavior as

   1. transference.

   2. counter-transference.

   3. identification.

   4. resistance.

7. A woman has remained close to the nurse all day. When the nurse talked with other clients during dinner, the client tried to regain the nurse's attention and then began to shout, "You're just like my mother. You pay attention to everyone but me!" The best interpretation of this behavior is that

   1. she is exhibiting resistance.

   2. she has been spoiled by her family.

   3. the nurse has failed to meet her needs.

   4. she is demonstrating transference.

8. A nurse is part of a community task force on teenage suicide. The task force is considering all of the following steps in an effort to reduce teen suicide. Which action represents primary prevention?

   1. Encourage emergency room staff to request psychiatric consultation for adolescents who overdose.

   2. Educate teachers, counselors, and school nurses in recognition and early intervention with suicidal teens.

   3. Provide community programs, such as Scouts, which increase self-esteem for children and adolescents.

   4. Increase the number of inpatient adolescent psychiatric beds available in the community.

9. Two nurses are discussing plans for their client group. What should be in the plan to promote group cohesiveness?

   1. Let the group know which clients are behaving in ways approved by the nurses.

   2. Help the group identify group goals that are consistent with the individual members' goals.

3. Make most decisions about the group in advance and make each group member aware of the nurses' decisions.

4. Seat the most talkative members nearest the nurses where they can be more clearly heard by the group.

10. The nurse is the leader of a client group. The members relate superficially, test each other and the group rules, and compete for the nurse's attention. This behavior is typical of which stage of group development?

   1. Orientation.
   2. Working.
   3. Feedback.
   4. Termination.

11. A family was referred to family therapy after their teenage son experienced behavioral problems in school. Which statement by the father indicates that he understands the purpose of family therapy?

   1. "Our son will realize the consequences of his actions and try harder to behave."
   2. "It will help us learn to communicate and problem solve better as a group."
   3. "I expect the therapist to tell my wife to quit babying our son."
   4. "The therapist will tell us how to make our son behave better in school."

12. A client walks in to the mental health outpatient center and states, "I've had it. I can't go on any longer. You've got to help me." The nurse asks the client to be seated in a private interview room. Which action should the nurse take next?

   1. Reassure the client that someone will help him soon.
   2. Assess the client's insurance coverage.
   3. Find out more about what is happening to the client.
   4. Call the client's family to come and provide support.

13. The nurse is caring for a client with anorexia nervosa who is to be placed on behavior modification. Which is appropriate to include in the nursing care plan?

   1. Remind the client frequently to eat all the food served on the tray.
   2. Increase phone calls allowed the client by one per day for each pound gained.
   3. Include the family with the client in therapy sessions 2 times per week.
   4. Weigh the client each day at 6:00 A.M. in hospital gown and slippers after she voids.

14. An adult is pacing about the unit and wringing his hands. He is breathing rapidly and complains of palpitations and nausea and he has difficulty focusing on what the nurse is saying. He says he is having a heart attack but refuses to rest. The nurse would interpret his level of anxiety as

    1. mild.
    2. moderate.
    3. severe.
    4. panic.

15. Each time a client is scheduled for a therapy session she develops headache and nausea. The nurse might interpret this behavior as

    1. conversion.
    2. reaction formation.
    3. projection.
    4. suppression.

16. A man is admitted to the intensive care unit with chest pain, an abnormal ECG, and elevated enzymes. When the significance of this is explained to him, he says, "I can't be having a heart attack. No way. You must be mistaken." The nurse suspects the client is using which defense mechanism?

    1. Sublimation.
    2. Regression.
    3. Dissociation.
    4. Denial.

17. An adult is admitted for panic attacks. He frequently experiences shortness of breath, palpitations, nausea, diaphoresis, and terror. What should the nurse include in the care plan when he is having a panic attack?

    1. Calm reassurance, deep breathing, and medication as ordered.
    2. Teach him problem solving in relation to his anxiety.
    3. Explain the physiologic responses of anxiety.
    4. Explore alternate methods for dealing with the cause of his anxiety.

18. A client on an inpatient psychiatric unit refuses to eat and states that the staff is poisoning her food. Which action should the nurse include in the client's care plan?

    1. Explain to the client that the staff can be trusted.
    2. Show the client that others eat the food without harm.
    3. Offer the client factory-sealed foods and beverages.
    4. Institute behavior modification with privileges dependent on intake.

19. A woman is being treated on the inpatient unit for depression. She tells the nurse, "I don't see how I can go on. I've been thinking of ways to kill myself. I can see several ways to do it." The best initial action for the nurse is to

   1. call the physician for orders.
   2. explain to the client the consequences of suicide on her family.
   3. see that someone is with the client at all times.
   4. help the client identify alternate means of coping.

20. An adult male has been admitted to the inpatient unit with a diagnosis of depression. He states that he continues to think of suicide and will be looking for a way to kill himself in the hospital. Which is most essential for the nurse to include in his nursing care plan?

   1. Encourage the client to participate in all unit activities.
   2. Explain to the client how suicide will affect his family.
   3. Allow the client time alone to relax and think.
   4. Have someone stay with the client 24 hours a day.

ANSWERS AND RATIONALES

1. 2. Negativism is common to the toddler in the anal stage of development (age 1 to 3) who is learning to assert his independence and mastery.

2. 4. Integrity includes acceptance of changes; a sense of continuity of past, present, and future; and acceptance of death.

3. 1. Preoperational-preconceptual children (5 to 7 years old) are learning to integrate concepts based on relationships and can comprehend the basic rules.

4. 1. The client needs orientation to the nurse and the situation. An open, honest approach in sharing these initial data will set the tone for the relationship.

5. 2. Many clients are anxious at the time of admission and are often reassured by a calm, competent professional approach, which should always be tried first. If the client is unable to respond to this, then other measures, such as medication, may be necessary.

6. 4. Resistance is characterized by conscious or unconscious actions that sabotage the relationship and thus help the client avoid confronting issues that may increase anxiety.

7. 4. Transference is the unconscious transfer of qualities originally associated with another relationship to the nurse. These are often qualities associated

with a parent or sibling and may provoke responses from the client that are not appropriate to the situation.

8. 3. Primary prevention involves making changes in the community that promote health and prevent disease.

9. 2. Goals that are best met by a group and that are consistent with the goals of the individual members foster cohesive groups.

10. 1. During the orientation phase, group members demonstrate these behaviors as they try to identify and develop trust with the group.

11. 2. Family therapy is aimed at improving communication and problem solving within the family group. The focus is on the family as a group, not on correcting the behavior of any one.

12. 3. The nurse must assess the client and his situation before the appropriate action can be determined.

13. 2. In behavior modification, rewards are tied to specific goals.

14. 4. Terror, physiologic changes, and inability to focus on the real world are characteristic of the most extreme form of anxiety, panic.

15. 1. Conversion changes anxious feelings into somatic symptoms.

16. 4. Denial helps the person escape unpleasant or intolerable reality by refusing to perceive the facts. It can serve as a normal protection in the early stages of crisis, but if the denial persists it will prevent the client from coping.

17. 1. Before any other interventions can be used, the client in panic must reduce his anxiety to a manageable level. The other interventions might be used when the client is less anxious.

18. 3. The client may be able to eat food that the staff has not handled.

19. 3. Maintaining client safety is the first priority. When a client is actively suicidal, one to one observation is necessary.

20. 4. The client who is actively suicidal needs constant observation to prevent him from carrying out his plan.

2

Psychiatric Disorders (DSM-IV-TR)

■ DISORDERS OF INFANCY, CHILDHOOD, AND ADOLESCENCE

Overview

A. A specific group of disorders beginning in infancy, childhood, or adolescence.
B. Clients in these age groups may also evidence other disorders such as depression or schizophrenia.
C. Intellectual, behavioral, and/or emotional dysfunction of the young client also has an effect on the family, which may require nursing intervention.

Assessment

Newborn/Infants

A. Maturation
B. Developmental level
C. Sensorimotor capabilities
D. Bonding
E. Response to cuddling

Children/Adolescents

A. Motor skills
B. Communication abilities
C. Vocational/academic skills
D. Social and behavioral problems
E. Behavioral changes
F. Growth and development: physical/emotional
G. Self-concept
H. Knowledge of disorder

Parent/Family

A. Response to infant/child/adolescent with disorder
B. Guilt, sense of loss
C. Sibling jealousy/resentment
D. Knowledge of disorder
E. Expectations
F. Plans for future (home care/institutionalization)

Analysis

Nursing diagnoses for a child/family with a psychiatric-mental health disorder may include

A. Client
　　1. Anxiety
　　2. Total incontinence
　　3. Ineffective coping
　　4. Risk for injury
　　5. Deficient knowledge
　　6. Deficient self-care
　　7. Low self-esteem
　　8. Disturbed sensory-perceptual
　　9. Sexual dysfunction
　　10. Risk for violence
B. Parents/family
　　1. Anxiety
　　2. Disabled family coping
　　3. Dysfunctional family process
　　4. Anticipatory grieving
　　5. Deficient knowledge
　　6. Impaired parenting

Planning and Implementation

Goals

A. Client will
　　1. Communicate thoughts and feelings about self-concept.
　　2. Perform tasks at optimal level of capability.
　　3. Develop trusting relationship with care givers.
B. Parents/family will
　　1. Communicate feelings and responses to child and to disorder.
　　2. Demonstrate knowledge of disorder.
　　3. Formulate plans for child's care.

Interventions

A. Client
1. Establish a therapeutic relationship by accepting client and client's limitations.
2. Promote communication by use of therapeutic techniques, play therapy.
3. Encourage independence in task performance with guidance and support.

B. Parents/family
1. Promote communication by accepting family responses.
2. Provide information about disorder.
3. Contact appropriate person/agency for consultation with family about care and assistance with the child.

Evaluation

Client

A. Demonstrates trust in care givers.
B. Relates feelings about self verbally or symbolically.
C. Performs activities of daily living (ADL) and tasks at optimal level.

Parents/Family

A. Relate positive/negative responses to child.
B. Demonstrate understanding of disorder and child's potential.
C. With consultant, formulate a plan for child's care.

Specific Disorders

Mental Retardation

Note: This is coded on Axis II.

A. General information
1. Significant subaverage intelligence (IQ of 70 or below) resulting in maladaptive behaviors with onset before age of 18 years
2. Etiology
    a. Heredity 5%
    b. Early alterations in embryonic development 30%
    c. Perinatal problems 10%
    d. Acquired in infancy/early childhood 5%
    e. Environmental/other mental disorders 15-20%
    f. Unknown etiology 30%-40%
3. Degrees of retardation
    a. Mild mental retardation (IQ 50-70)
        1) 85% of cases
        2) educable to 6th grade level
        3) able to become self-supporting

    b. Moderate mental retardation (IQ 35-49)
        1) 10% of cases
        2) educable to 2nd grade level
        3) able to perform skills but will need supervision at work
    c. Severe mental retardation (IQ 20-34)
        1) 3-4% of cases
        2) may learn to talk/communicate
        3) able to perform simple tasks and elementary hygiene
    d. Profound mental retardation (IQ below 20)
        1) 1-2% of cases
        2) some speech/communication possible

B. Assessment findings
    1. Intellectual impairment (determine degree)
    2. Sensorimotor impairment
    3. Communication, social, behavioral impairment
    4. Lack of self-esteem and poor self-image
    5. Sense of loss, guilt, nonacceptance or unrealistic expectations on part of parents/family

C. Nursing interventions
    1. Promote optimal functioning in ADL and feelings of accomplishment, self-worth.
    2. Provide opportunities for client/family to communicate thoughts, feelings.
    3. Provide positive reinforcement for every success.
    4. Accept client's limitations and set goals accordingly.
    5. Provide support and information about disorder to family.
    6. Accept family's response to client.

Other Disorders of Childhood/Adolescence

A. General information
    1. *Separation anxiety*: excessive anxiety and worry about being separated from person(s)/places to which child has become attached (e.g., refusal to leave mother/home to attend school)
    2. *Reactive/attachment disorder*: reluctance to enter social relationships with others, creating an interference with social growth
    3. *Overanxious disorders*: pervasive, unrealistic worry or concern about competency; somatic complaints without physical basis

B. Assessment findings: excessive anxiety related to separation, social interaction, and achievements

C. Nursing intervention: provide information regarding available mental health services for child and family.

Disorders with Physical Manifestations

A. General information
    1. Important to rule out any physiologic cause

    2. Often related to stress or conflict in the family

    3. May affect child's family/social interactions and development

B. Assessment findings

    1. *Enuresis*: urinary incontinence (bedwetting) after age 5 not caused by physical disorder

    2. *Encopresis*: fecal incontinence after age 4 not caused by physical disorder

    3. *Tics*: involuntary, repetitive movements

    4. *Stuttering*: repetition of sounds, words or frequent hesitations in speaking

C. Nursing interventions

    1. Provide information about the disorders and emphasize that they are treatable.

    2. Determine whether family therapy may be indicated, as well as individual therapy for child.

    3. Offer support and help child/family overcome feelings of shame or guilt.

    4. For enuresis and encopresis, utilize toilet training techniques.

    5. Encourage discussion of client/family response to symptoms.

■ PERVASIVE DEVELOPMENTAL DISORDERS

Autistic Disorder

A. General information

    1. Usually develops prior to 3 years of age.

    2. Child does not relate to people, but may become attached to objects.

    3. This is a rare disorder, may have a physiologic basis.

    4. Chronic disorder, more than $2/3$ of these children remain severely handicapped and dependent on caregivers.

    5. Special education is necessary.

    6. Family may choose institutionalization for optimum care.

B. Assessment findings

    1. Infant not responsive to cuddling; may even show an aversion to being touched

    2. No eye contact or facial responsiveness

    3. Impaired or no verbal communication

    4. Echolalia (repetition of words/phrases spoken by others)

    5. Inability to tolerate change

    6. Ritualistic behavior

    7. Fascination with movement, spinning objects

    8. Labile moods

    9. Unresponsive or overresponsive to stimuli

    10. High risk for developing seizure disorders

    11. Medications that have been used to assist in treatment of behavior are haloperidol, clomipramine, and SSRIs.

C. Nursing interventions
  1. Provide parents/family with support and information about the disorder, opportunities for therapy and education for the child.
  2. Assist child with ADL.
  3. Promote reality testing.
  4. Encourage child to develop a relationship with another person.
  5. Maintain regular schedule for activities.
  6. Provide constant routine for child (place for eating, sitting, sleeping).
  7. Protect child from self-injury.
  8. Provide safe environment.
  9. Institute seizure precautions if necessary.

Eating Disorders

A. General information
  1. Gross disturbances in eating behaviors
  2. *Pica*: persistent eating of substances such as plaster, paint, or sand
  3. *Bulimia nervosa*: binge eating; the ingestion of large amounts of food in short time, often followed by self-induced vomiting. May be accompanied by affective disorders and fear of being unable to stop this behavior. Manifested by fluctuations in weight caused by binges of eating and fasting. Antidepressant medications can be used in the treatment of bulimia.
  4. *Anorexia nervosa*: refusal to eat or aberration in eating patterns, resulting in severe emaciation that can be life threatening. Characterized by a fear of becoming fat, and a body-image disturbance where clients claim to feel fat even when extremely thin. This disorder is most common (95%) in adolescent and young adult females. There is a mortality rate of 7–18%. Antidepressant medications can be used in the treatment of anorexia.
B. Assessment findings (anorexia nervosa)
  1. Weight loss of 15% or more of normal body weight for age and height
  2. Electrolyte imbalance
  3. Depression
  4. Preoccupation with being thin; inability to recognize degree of own emaciation (distorted body image)
  5. Social withdrawal and poor family and individual coping skills
  6. History of high activity and achievement in academics, athletics
  7. Amenorrhea
C. Nursing interventions
  1. Monitor vital signs.
  2. Measure I&O.
  3. Weigh client 3 times/week at the same time (check to be sure client has not hidden heavy objects or water loaded before being weighed, weigh in hospital gown).

4. Do not comment on weight loss or gain.
5. Set limits on time allotted for eating.
6. Record amount eaten.
7. Stay with client during meals, focusing on client, not on food.
8. Accompany client to bathroom for at least ½ hour after eating to prevent self-induced vomiting.
9. Individual/family therapy may be necessary.
10. Encourage client to express feelings.
11. Help client to set realistic goal for self and to reduce need for being perfect.
12. Encourage client to discuss own body image; present reality; do not argue with client.
13. Teach relaxation techniques.
14. Help client identify interests and positive aspects of self.

■ DELIRIUM, DEMENTIA, AND OTHER COGNITIVE DISORDERS

Overview

A. A group of disorders with a known or presumed etiology.
B. Frequently manifest as dementia or delirium.
C. May be substance induced (drugs or alcohol) or caused by a disease process; etiology may be unknown.
D. It is important for the nurse to assess behaviors rather than focus on medical diagnoses.
E. Behaviors related to impaired brain functioning may be temporary or permanent, with increasing degeneration and eventual loss of brain function.
F. Not exclusive to old age, may complicate illnesses in any age group.

Types

A. *Delirium/Rapid Development*
   1. Manifested by reduced awareness of environment, disorders of perception, thought, speech, and attention deficits.
   2. Usually of brief duration.
   3. May occur postoperatively or following head injury, intoxication from drugs/alcohol, acute disease, or injury.
B. *Dementia/Gradual Development*
   1. Loss of intellectual abilities resulting in impaired social and occupational functioning.
   2. May be temporary, or progressive loss may occur.
   3. Found predominantly in elderly.
   4. Personality changes are usually an exaggeration of former character traits (e.g., suspicious, nontrusting person becomes paranoid); but

alteration can also occur (e.g., formerly neat and orderly person pays no attention to hygiene, becomes sloppy and dirty).

5. Memory impairment; short-term memory loss may be most obvious.
6. Organic etiology may be known; conditions include intoxication, infections, tumors, circulatory disorders (cerebral atherosclerosis), trauma, Huntington's chorea, Korsakoff's syndrome, Creutzfeld-Jakob disease, neurosyphilis.
7. Specific etiology may not be known (e.g., Alzheimer's disease, Pick's disease).
8. Frequently these clients cannot perform basic ADL.

Assessment

A. Mental status assessment, especially orientation to time and place, memory, and judgment
B. Nutritional status
C. Ability to perform ADL, self-care
D. Presence of confabulation (making up information to fill in memory gaps)
E. Behavioral/social changes
F. Disorders of perception
G. Impaired motor skills, coordination
H. Change in sleep patterns
I. Elimination: constipation/incontinence
J. Family response to client's condition

Analysis

Nursing diagnoses for clients with these disorders may include
A. Anxiety
B. Impaired verbal communication
C. Ineffective individual/family coping
D. Altered family processes
E. Risk for fluid volume deficit
F. Risk for injury
G. Imbalanced nutrition: less than body requirements
H. Self-care deficits
I. Low self-esteem
J. Disturbed sleep pattern
K. Disturbed thought processes
L. Risk for violence

Planning/Implementation

Goals

A. Client will
1. Be protected from injury.
2. Retain optimal cognitive function and self-care abilities.

3. Have fear/anxiety minimized.
4. Maintain adequate nutrition/hydration.

B. Family will communicate feelings about client.

Interventions

A. Institute safety measures: side rails, appropriate lighting in room, bed should be at lowest setting, frequent checks. Restraints should only be used as a last resort and for protection of client as ordered by physician and based on state and federal regulations.

B. Maintain reality orientation.
1. Client may not be capable of reality testing.
2. Continue to address client by name.
3. Maintain awareness of client's limitations in this area.
4. Do not tell client to "remember"; severe memory loss may make client incapable of memory.

C. Assist/support with self-care needs; arrange for necessary assistive devices, help with feeding; encourage fluids.

D. Avoid "insight" therapy and discussion of impaired mental functioning as this may increase anxiety.

E. Provide spouse/family with information about client's capabilities.

F. Provide support for spouse/family; encourage continued interaction with client.

G. Administer ordered medications (based on etiology), assess response, and provide education to the client and family. Medications might include short-acting benzodiazepines, antidepressants, cholinesterase inhibitors, or low-dose antipsychotics.

Evaluation

A. Client
1. Remains free from injuries.
2. Retains cognitive functions and self-care ability as far as possible; interacts with others appropriately.
3. Maintains appropriate weight.

B. Family
1. Expresses sense of loss or frustration related to client's condition.
2. Continues contact with client.

■ SUBSTANCE USE DISORDERS

Overview

A. The use of chemical agents (alcohol and drugs) to change behavior and mood

B. Abuse: continued use despite problems (social, occupational, psychologic) that are caused by substance or continued use in hazardous situations (e.g., operating machinery, driving)

NURSING ALERT

For the older adult, there is a greater risk for substance abuse related to altered mentation and increased usage of over-the-counter medications and prescription drugs. Loneliness is another factor. Substance abuse is frequently overlooked in this age group.

C. Dependence
   1. Need for larger amounts (tolerance)
   2. Unsuccessful attempts to decrease/ discontinue use
   3. Inability to function as usual in work, social activities
   4. Withdrawal symptoms (psychologic/ physical distress when substance is reduced/discontinued)
D. Addiction: compulsive use of a substance; physiologic and psychologic dependence

■ PSYCHOACTIVE SUBSTANCE-INDUCED ORGANIC MENTAL DISORDERS

The use of substances that result in intoxication or withdrawal syndromes, delirium, hallucinations, delusions, mood disorders.

Assessment

A. Determine substances used, amount and last time taken, and if combined with other drugs
B. Pupillary changes, changes in vital signs or level of consciousness
C. Presence of dehydration
D. Presence of nutritional and vitamin deficiencies
E. Suicide potential: ideation, gestures
F. Level of anxiety
G. Use of denial/projection
H. Symptoms of overdose (will be drug-specific; see Table 2-1)
I. Drug-use patterns: what, when, why substances are used

Analysis

Nursing diagnoses for clients with a psychoactive substance abuse disorder may include
A. Anxiety
B. Ineffective coping
C. Fear
D. Risk for fluid volume deficit
E. Risk for injury

TABLE 2-1 Commonly Abused Drugs

Drug	Effect	Dependence	Assessment Findings	Overdose	Nursing Interventions for Overdose
Barbiturates Antianxiety drugs, hypnotics	Reduction in anxiety, escape from stress	Psychologic at first, then physiologic; withdrawal similar to alcohol withdrawal, to point of delirium; cross-tolerance to other depressants	Irritability, weight loss, changes in mood or motor coordination	Slurred speech, lethargy, respiratory depression, coma; use combined with alcohol can be lethal	Keep person awake and moving to prevent coma; maintain airway.
Opioids/Narcotics Heroin, morphine, meperidine, methadone	Euphoria, dysphoria, and/ or apathy	Psychologic dependence rapidly leading to physical; signs of withdrawal: cramps, nausea, vomiting,	Pinpoint pupils, mental clouding, lethargy, impaired memory and judgment, evidence of needle tracks,	Depressed consciousness and respirations.. dilated pupils with anoxia or polydrug use	Provide emergency support of vital functions. In withdrawal, administer methadone or Narcan as ordered.

Stimulant		diarrhea; sleep disturbance, chills and shaking	inflamed nasal mucosa if drug is snorted		
Cocaine/Crack	Increased self-esteem, energy, sexual desire, euphoria; decreased anxiety	Dopamine deficiency results in psychologic dependency to produce feelings of well-being	Increased vital signs, headache, chest pain, depression and/or paranoia, inflamed nasal passages if snorted	Delirium, tremors, high fever (106+) convulsions, cardiac/respiratory arrest	Emergency support of vital functions, reduce CNS stimulation.
Amphetamines					
Amphetamine, dextroamphetamine, methamphetamine	Depressed appetite; increased activity, awareness, sense of well-being	Long-term use or high doses may produce delirium, paranoid-like delusions, withdrawal, depression, fatigue, sleep disturbances	Same as cocaine plus suicidal ideation	Same as cocaine,	Same as cocaine, plus suicide precautions. Observe for increased anxiety to panic, which may potentiate assaultive behavior.

Continued

Table 2-1 Continued

Drug	Effect	Dependence	Assessment Findings	Overdose	Nursing Interventions for Overdose
Phencyclidine (PCP)	Euphoria, psychomotor agitation, emotional lability	Not reported	Vomiting, hallucinations, paranoid ideation, agitation	Violent behavior, suicide, respiratory arrest, delirium, coma, increased blood pressure and pulse	Monitor vital signs. Observe for suicidal or assaultive behavior. Provide nonthreatening environment, reality orientation, support.
Hallucinogens LSD, mescaline	Disordered perceptions, depersonalization	Not reported	"Bad trip," high anxiety to panic;	Reduced LOC	Same as PCP, plus talk client down.

Cannabis Marijuana, hashish, THC	Euphoria, intense perceptions, relaxation, lethargy	Not reported	Increased pulse rate and appetite; impaired judgment and coordination	hallucinations may occur long after drug has been metabolized; flashbacks may produce long-lasting psychotic disorders	Panic reaction, nausea, vomiting, depression and disorders of perception	In panic, talk down. In severe depression, institute suicide precautions.

Continued

Table 2-1   Continued

Drug	Effect	Dependence	Assessment Findings	Overdose	Nursing Interventions for Overdose
Benzodiazepines Anti-anxiety drugs, muscle relaxants: clonazepam, diazepam, and others	Reduction in anxiety; anticonvulsant, reduces muscle spasms, reduces insomnia	Physical: dependence is low with oral dosing Psychologic: withdrawal syndrome may resemble an anxiety disorder Must differentiate withdrawal syndrome from anxiety disorders	Calm effect unless drug withdrawn abruptly Mild withdrawal including confusion, anterograde amnesia (impaired recall of events after dosing), anxiety, diaphoresis, tremors Effect may resemble alcohol intoxication	Mild sedation to stupor dependent on dose CNS depression, sedation to stupor, dose dependent Oral unlikely to cause significant respiratory depression without concomitant agents such as alcohol Intravenous may cause severe respiratory depression and death	Support vital body functions. Provide nonthreatening environment. Administer Narcan as ordered. Must be closely monitored.

F. Imbalanced nutrition: less than body requirements
G. Self-care deficit
H. Low self-esteem
I. Disturbed sensory-perceptual
J. Sleep deprivation
K. Disturbed thought processes
L. Risk for violence
M. Ineffective denial

Planning and Intervention

Goals

Client will
A. Be protected from injury.
B. Receive adequate hydration and nutrition.
C. Terminate use of substance being abused without withdrawal symptoms; emergency care will be provided if symptoms cannot be avoided.
D. Have decreased feelings of anxiety.
E. Receive information and consider help for substance-abuse disorder (e.g., AA or NA).

Interventions

A. Assess drug use pattern: identity, recent use, and frequency of use of prescription and nonprescription drugs, other substances (e.g., alcohol, nicotine).
B. Support client during acute phase of detoxification or withdrawal.
   1. Stay with client; reassure that current manifestations are temporary.
   2. Monitor vital signs, level of consciousness.
   3. Institute suicide precautions (if appropriate).
   4. Administer medications (to prevent withdrawal) as ordered.
   5. If client is experiencing panic, talk down, possibly with assistance of family/friends.
   6. If client is hallucinating, reinforce reality, speak in a calm voice.
   7. Confront client's use of denial.
   8. Monitor your own responses of sympathy/ anger.
   9. Be aware of transference/countertransference.
   10. Maintain course of action in plan of care; client must follow plan.
   11. Involve staff in negotiating care plan revisions.
C. Rehabilitation/longer-term care
   1. Provide nonthreatening environment.
   2. Set limits on unacceptable behavior.
   3. Provide adequate diet and fluids.
   4. Provide information relating to substance abuse and rehabilitation programs.

Evaluation

A. Client experienced no injury.
B. Vital signs are stable.
C. Withdrawal proceeded without symptoms; client remains drug/alcohol free.
D. Client can discuss substance-abuse problem and requests or agrees to consider rehabilitation/ therapy for problem.

Specific Disorders

Alcohol Abuse/Dependence

A. General information
   1. Alcohol is a legal substance and there are millions of social drinkers.
   2. Alcohol is classified as a central nervous system depressant.
   3. Alcohol abuse/dependence is a major problem in this country with over 18 million adults identified as alcohol abusers.
   4. Only approximately 5% of alcohol abusers are the "skid row" type.
   5. Incidence is increasing in women and adolescents.
   6. Considered a disease that can be arrested but not cured.
   7. Important to assess history of alcohol consumption for clients admitted to hospital for non-alcohol-related disorders, because they may go into withdrawal.
   8. Socioeconomic as well as a physiologic problem, resulting in increased health care costs and loss of productivity if ability to maintain a job is impaired.
   9. Alcohol used with other substances (barbiturates, antianxiety drugs) may have lethal consequences.
   10. Long-term use may result in loss of health (gastritis, pancreatitis, cirrhosis, hepatitis, malnutrition, cardiac and neural disorders) and life (suicide, automobile accidents).
   11. Directly related problems include withdrawal, delirium tremens, and alcohol-related dementia
      a. *Withdrawal*
         1) alcohol consumption reduced/ discontinued following continuous consumption for many days or longer
         2) withdrawal is progressive and has four stages:
            I. at least 8 hours after last drink; symptoms include mild tremors, tachycardia, increased blood pressure, diaphoresis, nervousness
            II. gross tremors, hyperactivity, profound confusion, loss of appetite, insomnia, weakness, disorientation, illusions, auditory and visual hallucinations
            III. 12–48 hours after last drink: symptoms include (in addition to those found in I and II) severe hallucinations, grand mal seizures

IV. 3-5 days after last drink (24-72 hours if untreated): delirium tremens, confusion, agitation, severe psychomotor activity, hallucinations, insomnia, tachycardia

3) withdrawal may last less than a week or may evolve into alcohol withdrawal delirium (delirium tremens).

4) 10-15% mortality rate from hypoglycemia/electrolyte imbalances.

b. *Delirium tremens (DTs)*

1) history of alcohol abuse usually for more than 5 years.

2) may be preceded by seizures.

3) symptoms occur 2-3 days after alcohol reduced/discontinued.

4) signs include tachycardia, increased blood pressure, agitation, delusions, hallucinations.

c. *Alcohol hallucinosis*: hallucinations only

d. *Alcohol-related dementia*: caused by poor nutrition

1) Korsakoff's psychosis is sometimes preceded by *Wernicke's encephalopathy.* Confusion and ataxia are predominant symptoms.

2) thiamine deficiency results in *Korsakoff's dementia/psychosis;* symptoms include chronic disorientation, confabulation. It is irreversible.

3) large doses of thiamine may prevent the development of Korsakoff's psychosis. See Table 2-2.

B. Medical management

1. Vitamin and nutrition therapy

2. Antianxiety drugs (Librium or Ativan)

3. Disulfiram (Antabuse)

a. Produces unpleasant reaction (thirst, sweating, palpitations, vomiting, dyspnea, respiratory and cardiac failure) when taken with alcohol.

b. 500 mg/day for 1-2 weeks; usual maintenance dose is 250 mg/day.

c. Duration of action is ½ to several hours; no alcohol should be taken at least 12 hours before taking drug.

d. Increases effects of antianxiety drugs and oral anticoagulants.

TABLE 2-2   Phases of Alcohol Addiction

Phase	Features
Prealcoholic	Drink almost every day to reduce tension Increase in amount of alcohol ingested
Addiction	Blackouts Secret drinking Large amounts ingested
Dependence	Physical craving for alcohol Makes up reasons for drinking Reduced nutrition Aggressive behavior Pressure from family and/or employer to reduce/stop drinking
Chronic	Long periods of intoxication Impaired thinking Less alcohol produces sedation tremors

      e. Side effects include headache, dry mouth, somnolence, flushing.
      f. Nursing responsibilities
         1) teach client the nature of severe reaction and importance of avoiding all alcohol (including cough medicine, foods prepared with alcohol, etc.).
         2) teach client to carry an identification card in case of accidental alcohol ingestion.
         3) monitor effects of antianxiety drugs if being taken at the same time.
         4) monitor for bleeding if taking oral anticoagulants.
   4. High doses of chlordiazepoxide (Librium) to control withdrawal in acute detoxification.
C. Assessment findings
   1. Dependent personality; often using denial as a defense mechanism
   2. Tendency to minimize and underreport amount of alcohol consumed
   3. Intoxication: blood alcohol level 0.15 (150 mg alcohol/100 ml blood). Legal level 0.08–0.10.
   4. Signs of impaired judgment, motor skills, and slurred speech
   5. Behavior may be boisterous and euphoric or aggressive, or may be depressed and withdrawn
   6. Signs of withdrawal, DTs, or alcohol-related dementias

DELEGATION TIP

nform family and support staff on how to encourage adequate nutritional intake for the client.

CLIENT TEACHING CHECKLIST

Educate the client and family about the following:

- Alcohol abuse triggers
- Support groups
- Adequate nutrition
- Alcohol abuse dependence and treatment

D. Nursing interventions
1. Stay with client.
2. Monitor vital signs and blood sugar levels.
3. Observe for tremors, seizures, increased agitation, anxiety, disorders of perception.
4. Administer medications as ordered; observe effects/side effects of tranquilizers carefully.
5. If disorders of perception occur, explain that these are part of the withdrawal process.
6. Provide fluids, adequate nutrition, and quiet environment.
7. When client is stable, provide information about rehabilitation programs (Alcoholics Anonymous); at this stage client may be willing to consider a program to stop drinking.
8. Provide information about Alanon (for spouse and adult family members), Alateen (for children), and ACOA (for adult children of alcoholics).

Psychoactive Drug Use

A. General information
1. Drugs abused may be prescription or "street" drugs
2. Types of drugs frequently abused
   a. Barbiturates, antianxiety drugs, hypnotics
   b. Opioids (narcotics): heroin, morphine, meperidine, methadone, hydromorphone

    c. Amphetamines: amphetamine, dextroamphetamine, methamphetamine (speed), some appetite suppressants

    d. Cocaine, hydrochloride cocaine (crack)

    e. Phencyclidine (PCP)

    f. Hallucinogens: LSD, mescaline, DMT

    g. Cannabis: marijuana, hashish, THC

B. Assessment findings and nursing interventions for overdoses vary with particular drug; see Table 2-1

C. Polydrug abusers

    1. Common pattern of drug use.

    2. Synergistic effect: drugs interact so that effect is greater than if each drug is taken separately.

    3. Additive effect: two or more drugs with same action are taken together (e.g., barbiturates with alcohol will result in heavy sedation).

Impaired Nurses

A. General information

    1. Most nursing licenses are suspended or revoked for substance abuse while on duty.

    2. Substances include alcohol and/or prescription drugs pilfered from unit drug stocks.

    3. Stealing drugs may result in criminal prosecution.

    4. Work-related stress and easy access to drugs are factors relating to nurses' substance abuse.

    5. Substance use results in impaired judgment and psychomotor abilities, resulting in unsafe nursing practice.

B. Assessment of impairment

    1. Alcohol odor on breath

    2. Frequent lateness/absences

    3. Shortages in narcotics

    4. Clients do not obtain pain relief after ''receiving'' pain reduction medication from nurse

    5. Nurse makes frequent trips to bathroom/locker room

    6. Changes in locomotion, psychomotor skills, pupil size, and mood/affect

C. Nurses' responsibilities related to impaired nurse colleague

    1. Client safety is first priority.

    2. ANA code of ethics (and most state laws) require nurse to safeguard clients.

    3. Interventions for suspected substance abuse by coworker

        a. Obtain information about legal issues, treatment options, and institutional policies.

        b. Document observations related to behaviors and narcotic charting.

    c. If possible, have other coworkers verify your information.

    d. Arrange meeting with peer(s), nurse, supervisor, nurse advocate (where possible) and confront nurse with documentation.

    e. Let nurse know you care about him/her and will help.

    f. Help nurse work through denial.

    g. Provide plan to offer recovery program (e.g., include "recovering" nurse buddy).

    h. Offer hope, support (moral and financial) to aid nurse in treatment.

    i. Explain institutional policies regarding future employment.

    j. If nurse continues to deny substance abuse, consider following steps
        1) advocate should protect nurse's rights.
        2) suspension/dismissal from job.
        3) report to licensing board.
        4) if theft of drug from unit has occurred, report to law enforcement agency.

■ SCHIZOPHRENIA AND OTHER PSYCHOTIC DISORDERS
Overview

A. Characterized by disordered thinking, delusions, hallucinations, depersonalization (feeling of being strange, not oneself), impaired reality testing (psychosis), and impaired interpersonal relationships.

B. Regression to the earliest stages of development is often noted (e.g., incontinence, mutism).

C. Onset is usually in adolescence/early adulthood (15 to 35 years of age).

D. Client may be seriously impaired and unable to perform ADL.

E. Etiology is not known; theories include
    1. Genetic: 1% of population.
    2. Biochemical: neurotransmitter dysfunction i.e., dopamine, serotonin.
    3. Interaction of predisposing risk and environmental stress.

F. Prior to onset (premorbid) client may have been suspicious, eccentric, or withdrawn.

Classifications

A. *Disorganized*: incoherent; delusions are not organized; social withdrawal; affect blunted, silly, or inappropriate

B. *Catatonic*: psychomotor disturbances
    1. Stupor: mute, little reaction or movement
    2. Excitement: purposeless, excited motor activity
    3. Posturing: voluntary, inappropriate, bizarre postures

C. *Paranoid*: delusions and hallucinations of persecution/grandeur

D. *Undifferentiated*: disorganized behaviors, delusions, and hallucinations

Assessment

A. Four As
1. Affect: flat, blunted
2. Associative looseness: verbalizations are disorganized
3. Ambivalence: cannot choose between conflicting emotions
4. Autistic thinking: thoughts on self, extreme withdrawal, unable to relate to outside world
B. Any changes in thoughts, speech, affect
C. Ability to perform self-care activities, nutritional deficits
D. Suicide potential
E. Aggression
F. Regression
G. Impaired communication

Analysis

Nursing diagnoses for clients with schizophrenic disorders may include
A. Anxiety
B. Impaired verbal communication
C. Ineffective coping
D. Risk for injury
E. Imbalanced nutrition: less than body requirements
F. Powerlessness
G. Self-care deficit
H. Low self-esteem
I. Disturbed sensory-perceptual
J. Disturbed sleep pattern
K. Social isolation
L. Risk for violence

Planning and Implementation

Goals

Client will
A. Develop a trusting/therapeutic relationship with nurse.
B. Be oriented, able to test reality.
C. Be protected from injury.
D. Be able to recognize impending loss of control.
E. Adhere to medication regimen.
F. Participate in activities.
G. Increase ability to care for self.

Interventions

A. Offer self in development of therapeutic relationship.
B. Use silence.

C. Set time for interaction with client.
D. Encourage reality orientation but understand that delusions/hallucinations are real to client.
E. Assist with feeding/dressing as necessary.
F. Check on client frequently, remove potentially harmful objects.
G. Contract with client to tell you when anxiety is becoming so high that loss of control is possible.
H. Administer antipsychotic medications as ordered (see Table 2-3 for side effects and dosages); observe for effects.
1. Reduction of hallucinations, delusions, agitation
2. Postural hypotension
    a. Obtain baseline blood pressure and monitor sitting/standing.
    b. Client must lie prone for 1 hour following injection.
    c. Teach client to sit up or stand up slowly.
    d. Elevate client's legs while seated.
    e. Withhold drug if systolic pressure drops more than 20–30 mmHg from previous reading.
3. Photosensitivity
    a. Advise use of sun screen.
    b. Avoid exposure to sunlight.
4. Agranulocytosis
    a. Instruct client to report sore throat or fever.
    b. Institute reverse isolation if necessary.
5. Elimination
    a. Measure I&O.
    b. Check bladder distention.
    c. Keep bowel record.
6. Sedation
    a. Avoid use of heavy machinery.
    b. Do not drive.
7. Extrapyramidal symptoms (EPs)
    a. Dystonic reactions
        1) sudden contractions of face, tongue, throat, extraocular muscles
        2) administer antiparkinson agents prn (e.g., benztropine [Cogentin] 1–8 mg or diphenhydramine [Benadryl] 10–50 mg), which can be given PO or IM for faster relief; trihexyphenidyl [Artane] 3–15 mg PO only, can also be used prn).
        3) remain with client; this is a frightening experience and usually occurs when medication is started.
    b. Parkinson syndrome
        1) occurs within 1–3 weeks
        2) tremors, rigid posture, masklike facial appearance
        3) administer antiparkinson agents prn.

TABLE 2-3 Antipsychotic Medications

Drug Classification	Dosages			Significant Side Effects
	Acute Symptoms	Maintenance/Day	Range/Day	
Chlorpromazine (Thorazine)	25–100 mg IM q1–4h prn	200–600 mg PO	25–2000 mg PO	Sedation Anticholinergic effects: dry mouth, blurred vision, constipation, urinary retention, postural hypotension
Fluphenazine HCl (Prolixin)	1.25 mg IM, max 10 mg IM, divided doses	1–5 mg PO	1–30 mg PO	Extrapyramidal effects
Fluphenazine decanoate/enanthate (Prolixin)	–	25 mg IM q2wk	25–100 mg IM	Extrapyramidal
Trifluoperazine (Stelazine)	1–2 mg IM q4h; 2–4 mg PO, max 10 mg qd	2–4 mg PO	2–80 mg PO	Extrapyramidal
Haloperidol (Haldol)	2–10 mg IM in divided doses	2–8 mg PO	1–100 mg PO	Extrapyramidal

Drug				Side effects
Thiothixene (Navane)	8-16 mg IM in divided doses	6-10 mg PO	6-60 mg PO	Extrapyramidal
Loxapine (Loxitane)	-	60-100 mg PO	30-250 mg PO	Extrapyramidal
Olanzapine (Zyprexa)	10-20 mg PO	5-20 mg PO	2.5-20 mg PO	Sedation, weight gain, increased glucose and lipid levels
Quetepine (Seroquel)	400-800 mg PO	200-600 mg PO	25-800 mg PO	Sedation, may accelerate cataract formation
Ziprasidone (Geodon)	40-80 mg PO BID with food or 10-20 mg IM BID	20-80 mg PO BID	20-80 mg PO BID 10-40 mg IM	Nausea, anxiety, insomnia (transient); QTC prolongation
Aripiprazole (Abilify)	15-30 mg PO	15-30 mg PO	15-30 mg PO	Nausea, insomnia
Clozapine (Clozaril)	-	300-450 mg PO	75-700 mg PO	Agranulocytosis; sedation
Risperidone (Risperdal)	2-6 mg PO	2-6 mg PO	0.25 mg-8 mg PO	Increased prolactin levels, EPS at higher doses, sedation

    c. Akathisia
        1) motor restlessness
        2) need to keep moving
        3) administer antiparkinson agents.
        4) do not mistake this for agitation; do not increase antipsychotic medication.
        5) reduce medications to see if symptoms decrease.
        6) determine if movement is under voluntary control.
    d. Tardive dyskinesia
        1) irreversible involuntary movements of tongue, face, extremities
        2) may occur after prolonged use of antipsychotics
    e. Neuroleptic malignant syndrome
        1) occurs days/weeks after initiation of treatment in 1% of clients
        2) elevated vital signs, rigidity, and confusion followed by incontinence, mutism, opisthotonos, retrocollis, renal failure, coma, and death
        3) discontinue medication, notify physician, monitor vital signs, electrolyte balance, I&O
    f. Elderly clients should receive doses reduced by one-half to one-third of recommended level
I. Encourage participation in milieu, group, art, and occupational therapies when client able to tolerate them.

Evaluation

Client
A. Stays with nurse prescribed period of time.
B. Is oriented to reality, can state name, place, and date.
C. Can feed/dress self with specified amount of assistance.
D. Has not attempted/will not attempt to injure self or others.
E. Adheres to medication regimen with minimal side effects.
F. Participates in activities.

■ MOOD DISORDERS

Overview

A. Characterized by disturbance in mood (affect) that is either depression or elation (mania); occur in a variety of patterns, alone or together (see Figure 2-1). Disturbance is beyond normal range of mood experienced by most people.
B. *Bipolar disorder:* components of both depression and elation (formerly called manic-depression)
C. *Cyclothymic disorder:* milder symptoms of both mania and depression, often separated by long periods of normal mood

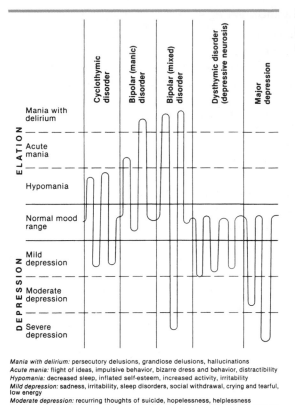

FIGURE 2-1   Patterns of mood disturbances in affective disorders

Mania with delirium: persecutory delusions, grandiose delusions, hallucinations
Acute mania: flight of ideas, impulsive behavior, bizarre dress and behavior, distractibility
Hypomania: decreased sleep, inflated self-esteem, increased activity, irritability
Mild depression: sadness, irritability, sleep disorders, social withdrawal, crying and tearful, low energy
Moderate depression: recurring thoughts of suicide, hopelessness, helplessness
Severe depression: delusions, hallucinations, psychomotor retardation and stupor, agitation (in depression with melancholia)

D. *Dysthymic disorder:* long-standing symptoms of depression alternating with short periods of normal mood; client usually able to maintain roles in job, school, etc.

E. Etiology is unknown; theories include
  1. Genetic: approximately 7% of general population; risk is 20% if a close relative has depression
  2. Biochemical: dysregulation in norepinephrine and serotonin
  3. Psychoanalytic: anger turned inward (i.e., anger toward significant other is turned into anger toward self)

Assessment

A. Mood: dysphoric; blue/sad or elated/aggressive
B. Presence of psychomotor agitation, retardation, or hyperactivity
C. Disorders of cognition: narrowed perception and interests, impaired concentration, grandiose delusions, flight of ideas in elation stage
D. Sexual functioning changes

E. Appropriateness of appearance/dress
F. Appetite
G. Potential for suicide

Analysis

Nursing diagnoses for clients with affective disorders may include
A. Constipation
B. Impaired verbal communication
C. Ineffective coping
D. Risk for injury
E. Imbalanced nutrition: less than body requirements
F. Self-care deficit
G. Disturbed self-esteem
H. Disturbed sleep pattern
 I. Disturbed thought processes

Planning and Implementation

Goals

Client will
A. Be protected from injury.
B. Receive adequate rest and sleep.
C. Maintain adequate intake of fluids and nutrients, regular elimination.
D. Develop trusting/therapeutic relationship with nurse.
E. Be oriented to reality.
F. Participate in planned activities.

Interventions

A. Assess for suicide potential.
B. Encourage verbalization of feelings of hopelessness and helplessness.
C. Provide quiet environment for rest and sleep.
D. Provide small, attractive meals; encourage intake of fluids.
E. Maintain bowel record.
F. Use silence and broad openings, focus on client's verbal/nonverbal behaviors.
G. Present reality but accept client's need for delusions.
H. Accept client's negative responses, hostility.
 I. Provide activities and tasks to raise client's self-esteem.
J. Assist with self-care as needed.
K. If client is agitated
   1. Work with client on a one-to-one basis.
   2. Walk with client; provide some diversional activity.
   3. Reduce environmental stimuli (e.g., put in a quiet room, dim lights).

Evaluation

Client

A. Has gained or maintained weight.
B. Reports any suicidal ideation.
C. Sleeps a specified number of hours.
D. Can meet own needs for ADL.
E. Has realistic appraisal of self.

Specific Disorders

Bipolar Disorder (Manic Episode)

A. General information
  1. Onset usually before age 30
  2. Characterized by hyperactivity and euphoria that may become sarcasm or hostility
B. Assessment findings
  1. Hyperactivity to the point of physical exhaustion
  2. Flamboyant dress/makeup
  3. Sexual acting out
  4. Impulsive behaviors
  5. Flight of ideas: inability to finish one thought before jumping to another
  6. Loud, domineering, manipulative behavior
  7. Distractibility
  8. Dehydration, nutritional deficits
  9. Delusions of grandeur
  10. Possible short-term depression (risk of suicide)
  11. Hostility, aggression
C. Medical management
  1. Lithium carbonate (Eskalith, Lithobid, Lithotabs)
     a. Initial dosage levels: 600 mg TID, to maintain a blood serum level of 1.0-1.5 mEq/liter; blood serum levels should be checked 12 hours after last dose, twice a week.
     b. Maintenance dosage levels: 300 mg TID/QID, to maintain a blood serum level of 0.4-1.0 mEq/liter; checked monthly.
     c. Toxicity when blood levels higher than 2.0 mEq/liter: tremors, nausea and vomiting, thirst, polyuria, coma, seizures, cardiac arrest
  2. Antipsychotics may also be given for hyperactivity, agitation, psychotic behavior. Chlorpromazine (Thorazine) and haloperidol (Haldol) are most commonly used (see Table 2-3).
D. Nursing interventions
  1. Determine what client is attempting to tell you; use active listening.
  2. Assist client in focusing on a topic.

3. Offer finger foods, high-nutrition foods, and fluids.
4. Provide quiet environment, decrease stimuli.
5. Stay with client, use silence.
6. Remove harmful objects.
7. Be accepting of hostile statements.
8. Do not argue with client.
9. Use distraction to divert client from behaviors that are harmful to self or others.
10. Administer medications as ordered and observe for effects/side effects.
    a. Teach clients early signs of toxicity.
    b. Maintain fluid and salt intake.
    c. Avoid diuretics.
    d. Monitor lithium blood levels.
11. Assist in dressing, bathing.
12. Set limits on disruptive behaviors.

Major Depression

A. General information
   1. Characterized by loss of ambition, lack of interest in activities and sex, low self-esteem, and feelings of boredom and sadness.
   2. Etiology may be physiologic or response to an actual or perceived loss.
   3. These clients are at high risk for suicide, especially when depressed mood begins to lift and/or energy level increases.
B. Medical management
   1. Tricyclic antidepressants: amitriptyline HCl, etc.; see Table 2-4
   2. Monoamine oxidase inhibitors (MAOIs): isocarboxazid (Marplan), etc.; see Table 2-4
   3. Atypical antidepressants: fluoxetin (Prozac), sertraline (Zoloft), etc.
   4. Electroconvulsive therapy (ECT)
C. Assessment findings
   1. Feelings of helplessness, hopelessness, worthlessness
   2. Reduction in normal activities or agitation
   3. Slowing of body functions/elimination
   4. Loss of appetite
   5. Inappropriate guilt
   6. Self-deprecation, low self-esteem
   7. Inability to concentrate, disordered thinking
   8. Poor hygiene
   9. Slumped posture
   10. Crying, ruminating (relates same incident over and over)
   11. Dependency
   12. Depressed children: possible separation anxiety

TABLE 2-4   Antidepressant Medications

Drug	Initiating	Dosage Maintenance	Side Effects
SSRIs Fluoxetine (Prozac) (Prozac Weekly)	20 mg PO	20–40 mg/day or 90 mg once per week (once stable)	Sexual dysfunction; nausea, diarrhea, HA, anxiety (transient)
Sertraline (Zoloft)	50 mg PO	50–200 mg/ day	As above
Paroxetine (Paxil) (Paxil CR)	20 mg PO 25 mg PO	20–40 mg/day 25–50 mg/day	As above
Citalopram (Celexa)	20 mg PO	20–80 mg/day	Sexual dysfunction; nausea, HA, nervousness (transient)
Escitalopram (Lexapro)	10 mg PO	10–20 mg/day	As above
Fluvoxamine (Luvox)	50 mg PO HS	50–300 mg HS	Tiredness, sexual dysfunction; HA, nausea, nervousness (transient) (used in treatment of OCD)
Atypical Antidepressants: Bupropion (Wellbutrin SR)	100 mg PO	150 mg BID	Anxiety, insomnia; can lower seizure threshold in overdose
Mirtazapine (Remeron)	15 mg PO HS	30–45 mg HS	Sedation at 15 mg (less at higher doses); increased appetite
Nefazodone (Serzone)	50 mg PO HS	50–600 mg HS	Sedation, dry mouth, postural hypotension; liver toxicity

Continued

Table 2-4   Continued

Drug	Initiating	Dosage Maintenance	Side Effects
Venlafaxine (Effexor XR)	37.5 mg PO	75–375 mg	Sexual dysfunction; HA, nausea, nervousness; can increase BP at doses > 300 mg/day
Trazodone (Desyrel)	150 mg PO in divided doses	150–400 mg PO in divided doses	Sedation, anxiety, hypotension, priapism (commonly used as sleep aid)
Tricyclics Amitriptyline (Elavil, Endep)	75–100 mg PO	50–150 mg PO at bedtime; 80–100 mg IM in divided doses	Constipation, blurred vision, drowsiness, orthostatic hypotension, urinary retention, dry mouth, increased appetite, sexual dysfunction
Clomipramine (Anafranil)	75–250 mg PO in divided doses at HS	50–150 mg PO at HS	As above
Desipramine (Norpramin)	50 mg HS	100–150 mg HS	As above
Nortriptyline	50 mg HS	50–125 mg HS	As above
Monoamine Oxidase Inhibitors (MAOIs) Isocarboxazid (Marplan)	30 mg PO in divided doses	10–30 mg PO	As for tricyclics, plus angina, hypoglycemia, hypertensive crisis precipitated by ingestion of foods with tyramine or concurrent use of tricyclics
Phenalizine (Nardil)	60 mg PO in divided doses	30–60 mg PO	As above

13. Elderly clients: possible symptoms of dementia
14. Somatic and persecutory delusions and hallucinations
D. Nursing interventions
  1. Monitor I&O.
  2. Weigh client regularly.
  3. Maintain a schedule of regular appointments.
  4. Remove potentially harmful articles.
  5. Contract with client to report suicidal ideation, impulses, plans; check client frequently.
  6. Assist with dressing, hygiene, and feeding.
  7. Encourage discussion of negative/positive aspects of self.
  8. Encourage change to more positive topics if self-deprecating thoughts persist.
  9. Administer antidepressant medications (see Table 2-4) as ordered.
    a. Tricyclic antidepressants (TCAs)
      1) effectiveness increased by antihistamines, alcohol, benzodiazepines
      2) effectiveness decreased by barbiturates, nicotine, vitamin C
    b. Monoamine oxidase inhibitors (MAOIs)
      1) effectiveness increased with anti-psychotic drugs, alcohol, meperidine
      2) avoid foods containing tyramine (e.g., beer, red wine, aged cheese, avocados, caffeine, chocolate, sour cream, yogurt); these foods or MAOIs taken with TCAs may result in hypertensive crisis.
    c. Be sure client swallows medication. If side effects disappear suddenly, cheeking/ hoarding may have occurred. These medications can be used to attempt suicide.
    d. Antidepressant medications do not take effect for 2-3 weeks. Encourage client to continue medication even if not feeling better. Be aware of suicide potential during this time.
    e. Warn client not to take any drugs without consulting physician.
  10. Assist with ECT as ordered.
    a. Give normal pre-op preparation, including informed consent.
    b. Remove all hairpins, dentures.
    c. Ensure client is wearing loose clothing.
    d. Check vital signs after the procedure.
    e. Reorient and assure that any memory loss is temporary.
    f. Assist to room or to care of responsible party if outpatient.

Dysthymic Disorder

A. General information: chronic mood disturbance of at least 2 years' duration for adults, 1 year for children
B. Assessment findings
   1. Normal moods for a period of weeks, followed by depression
   2. Insomnia/hypersomnia
   3. Social withdrawal
   4. Loss of interest in activities
   5. Recurrent thoughts of suicide and death
C. Nursing interventions: same as for major depression.

■ NEUROTIC DISORDERS

In DSM-IV-TR, the disorders formerly categorized as neurotic disorders are included in Anxiety, Somatoform, and Dissociative Disorders. Reality testing is intact.

■ ANXIETY DISORDERS

Overview

A. Common element is anxiety, manifested in a variety of behaviors.
B. Therapy relates to reduction of anxiety; when anxiety is reduced, the symptoms will be alleviated.
C. Types include generalized anxiety disorder, panic disorder, phobic disorders, and obsessive-compulsive disorders.

Assessment

A. Level of anxiety: may be to point of panic
B. Vital signs: may be elevated
C. Reality testing: should be intact; can recognize that thoughts are irrational but cannot control them
D. Physical symptoms: no organic basis
E. Memory: possible memory loss or loss of identity
F. Pattern of symptoms: chronic with a pattern of waxing and waning or sudden onset

Analysis

Nursing diagnoses for the client with an anxiety disorder may include
A. Anxiety
B. Fear
C. Ineffective coping
D. Powerlessness
E. Deprivation of sleep
F. Disturbed thought processes

Planning and Implementation

Goals

Client will
A. Develop a trusting/therapeutic relationship with nurse.
B. Recognize causes of anxiety and develop alternative coping mechanisms.
C. Reduce/alleviate symptoms of anxiety.

Interventions

A. Encourage discussion of anxiety and relationship to symptoms.
B. Provide calm, accepting atmosphere.
C. Administer antianxiety medications (for short-term use only) as ordered and monitor effects/side effects.
    1. Diazepam (Valium): 5-20 mg PO daily; 2-10 mg IM or IV daily
    2. Chlordiazepoxide (Librium): 20-100 mg PO daily; 50-100 mg IM or IV daily
    3. Alprazolam (Xanax) 0.75-4 mg PO daily
    4. Oxazepam (Serax) 30-120 mg PO daily
    5. Triazolam (Halcion) 0.25-0.5 mg HS
    6. Side effects
        a. Client may become addicted.
        b. Additive effect with alcohol.
        c. Dizziness may occur when treatment initiated.
        d. Lower doses for elderly client.
        e. Do not stop abruptly; taper doses.
D. Teach client about self-medication regimen and side effects.

Evaluation

Client
A. Can discuss causes of anxiety with nurse.
B. Demonstrates constructive coping mechanisms and ability to reduce anxiety.
C. Demonstrates knowledge of effects and hazards of antianxiety medications.

Specific Disorders

Phobic Disorders

A. General information
    1. Irrational fears resulting in avoidance of objects or situations.
    2. Repressed conflicts are projected to outside world and eventually are displaced onto an object or situation.

3. Client can recognize that fear of these objects/situations is irrational, but cannot control emotional response when confronting or thinking about confronting the particular object/situation.

B. Assessment findings
   1. *Agoraphobia*: most serious phobia; fear of being alone or in public places; may reach point where client panics at thought of being in public places and cannot leave home.
   2. *Social phobias*: fear of being in situations where one may be scrutinized and embarrassed by others.
   3. *Specific phobias*: irrational fear of specific objects/situations (e.g., snakes, insects, heights, closed places).

C. Nursing interventions
   1. Know that behavior modification and systematic desensitization most commonly used; client cannot be "reasoned" out of behavior.
   2. Do not force contact with feared object/situation; may result in panic.
   3. Administer benzodiazepines (alprazolam or clonazepam), SSRIs, venlafaxine, or buspirone as ordered.
   4. Instruct in and encourage use of relaxation techniques.

Generalized Anxiety Disorder

A. General information
   1. Persistent anxiety for at least 1 month
   2. Cannot be controlled by client or displaced, remains free-floating and diffuse

B. Assessment findings
   1. Motor tensions: trembling, muscle aches, jumpiness
   2. Autonomic hyperactivity: sweating, palpitations, dizziness, upset stomach, increased pulse and respirations
   3. Affect: worried and fearful of what might happen
   4. Hyperalert: insomnia, irritability

C. Nursing interventions
   1. Stay with client.
   2. Encourage discussion of anxiety and its source.
   3. Provide calm, relaxing atmosphere.
   4. Administer antianxiety drugs, as ordered.
   5. Observe for effects and side effects.
   6. Monitor vital signs.
   7. Assess for level of anxiety.

Panic Disorder (with/without Agoraphobia)

A. General information: acute, panic-like attack lasting from a few minutes to an hour.

B. Assessment findings
   1. Sudden onset of intense fear/terror

2. Symptoms: include dyspnea, palpitations, chest pain, sensation of smothering or choking, faintness, fear of dying, dizziness
3. When severe, symptoms mimic acute cardiac disease that must be ruled out.
4. Client may be seen in ER.
C. Nursing interventions: same as for generalized anxiety disorder.

Obsessive-Compulsive Disorder (OCD)

A. General information
1. *Obsession*
   a. Recurrent thoughts that client cannot control; often violent, fearful, or doubting in nature (e.g., fear of contamination).
   b. Client cannot keep thoughts from intruding into consciousness; eventually resort to defense of undoing (performing ritual behavior).
2. *Compulsion*
   a. Action (ritual behavior) that serves to reduce tension from obsessive thought.
   b. Client may not desire to perform behavior but is unable to stop, as this is the only relief from distress.
   c. May interfere with social/occupational functioning.
B. Nursing interventions
1. Allow compulsive behavior, but set reasonable limits.
2. Permit client to complete behavior once started; aggression may result if behavior is not allowed or completed.
3. Engage client in alternative behaviors (client will not be able to do this alone).
4. Provide opportunities to perform tasks that meet need for perfectionism (e.g., stacking and folding linens).
5. As compulsive behavior decreases, help client to verbalize feelings, concerns.
6. Help client to make choices, participate in decisions regarding own schedule.
7. Administer clomipramine (Anafranil) as ordered. Gradual decrease in symptoms may take 2–3 months. Often used with behavior modification therapy (see Table 2-4).

Post-Traumatic Stress Disorder (PTSD)

A. General information
1. Disturbed/disintegrated response to significant trauma
2. Symptoms can occur following crisis event such as war, earthquake, flood, airplane crash, rape, or assault
3. Reexperiencing of traumatic event in recollections, nightmares

B. Assessment findings
1. Psychic numbing: not as responsive to persons and events as to the traumatic experience
2. Sleep disturbances (e.g., nightmares)
3. Avoidance of environment/activities likely to arouse recall of trauma
4. Symptoms of depression
5. Possible violent outbursts
6. Memory impairment
7. Panic attacks
8. Substance abuse
C. Nursing interventions
1. Arrange for individual or group psychotherapy with others who experienced same trauma (e.g., Vietnam war veterans).
2. Provide crisis counseling, family therapy as needed.
3. Provide referrals.

■ SOMATOFORM DISORDERS

Overview

A. Anxiety is manifested in somatic (physical) symptoms.
B. There is organic pathology but no organic etiology.
C. Symptoms are real and not under voluntary control of the client.
D. Defense used is somatization or conversion: anxiety is transformed to a physical symptom.

Specific Disorders

Somatization Disorder

A. General information
1. Multiple, recurrent somatic complaints (fatigue, backache, nausea, menstrual cramps) over many years
2. No organic etiology for these complaints
B. Assessment findings
1. Complaints chronic but fluctuating
2. History of seeking medical attention for many years
3. Symptoms of anxiety and depression
4. Somatic complaints may involve any organ system
C. Nursing interventions
1. Be aware of own response (irritation/ impatience) to client.
2. Rule out organic basis for current complaints.
3. Focus on anxiety reduction, not physical symptoms.
4. Minimize secondary gain.

Conversion Disorder

A. General information
1. Sudden onset of impairment or loss of motor or sensory function.
2. No physiologic cause.
3. Defenses used are repression and conversion; anxiety is converted to a physical symptom.
4. Temporal relationship between distressing event and development of symptom (e.g., unconscious desire to hit another may produce paralysis of arm).
5. Primary gain: client is not conscious of conflict. Anxiety is converted to a symptom that removes client from anxiety-producing situation.
6. Secondary gain: gain support and attention that was not previously provided. Tends to encourage client to maintain symptoms.
B. Assessment findings
1. Sudden paralysis, blindness, deafness, etc.
2. "La belle indifférence": inappropriately calm when describing symptoms
3. Symptoms not under voluntary control
4. Usually short term; symptoms will abate as anxiety diminishes
C. Nursing interventions
1. Focus on anxiety reduction, not physical symptom.
2. Use matter-of-fact acceptance of symptom.
3. Encourage client to discuss conflict.
4. Do not provide secondary gain by being too attentive.
5. Provide diversionary activities.
6. Encourage expression of feelings.

Pain Disorder

A. General information: complaint of severe and prolonged pain
B. Assessment findings
1. Pain impairs social/occupational function
2. Pain often severe
3. Sleep may be interrupted by experience of pain
C. Nursing interventions
1. Pain management
2. Encourage participation in activities

Hypochondriasis

A. General information
1. Unrealistic belief of having serious illnesses.
2. Belief persists despite medical reassurance.
3. Defenses used are regression and somatization.
B. Assessment findings

    1. Preoccupation with bodily functions, which are misinterpreted.
    2. History of seeing many doctors, many diagnostic tests.
    3. Dependent behavior: desires/demands great deal of attention.

C. Nursing interventions
    1. Rule out presence of actual disease.
    2. Focus on anxiety, not physical symptom.
    3. Set limits on amount of time spent with client.
    4. Reduce anxiety by providing diversionary activities.
    5. Avoid negative response to client's demands by discussing in staff conferences.
    6. Provide client with correct information.

■ DISSOCIATIVE DISORDERS

Overview

A. Sudden change in client's consciousness, identity, or memory.
B. Loss of memory, knowledge of identity, or how individual came to be in a particular place.
C. Defenses are repression and dissociation.

Specific Disorders

Dissociative Amnesia

A. General information: inability to recall information about self with no organic reason
B. Assessment findings
    1. No history of head injury
    2. Retrograde amnesia, may extend far into past
C. Nursing interventions
    1. Rule out organic causes.
    2. Reassure client that his/her identity will be made known to him/her.
    3. Provide safe environment.
    4. Establish nurse-client relationship to reduce anxiety.

Dissociative Fugue

A. General information
    1. Client travels to strange, often distant place; unaware of how he traveled there, and unable to recall past.
    2. May follow severe psychologic stress.
B. Assessment findings
    1. Memory loss
    2. May have assumed new identity
    3. No recall of fugue state when normal functions return
C. Nursing interventions: same as for psychogenic amnesia.

■ PERSONALITY DISORDERS

Note: This is coded on Axis II.

Overview

A. Patterns of thinking about self and environment become maladaptive and cause impairment in social or occupational functioning or subjective distress.

B. Usually develop by adolescence.

C. Most common is borderline personality disorder.

Specific Disorders

Borderline Personality Disorder

A. General information: clients are impulsive and unpredictable, have difficulty interacting; characterized by behavior problems

B. Assessment findings
1. Unstable, intense interpersonal relationships
2. Impulsive, unpredictable, manipulative behavior; prone to self-harm
3. Marked mood shifts from anger to dysphoric
4. Uncertainty about self-image, gender identity, values
5. Chronic intolerance of being alone, feelings of boredom
6. Splitting: distinct separation of love and hate; views others as *all* good or *all* bad.
7. Use of projection and regression

C. Nursing interventions
1. Protect from self-mutilation, suicidal gestures.
2. Establish therapeutic relationship, be aware of own responses to manipulative behaviors.
3. Maintain objectivity.
4. Use a calm approach.
5. Set limits.
6. Apply plan of care consistently.
7. Interact with clients when they demonstrate appropriate behavior.
8. Teach relaxation techniques.

Antisocial Personality Disorder

A. General information
1. Chronic history of antisocial behaviors (e.g., fighting, stealing, aggressive behaviors, substance abuse, criminal behaviors).
2. These behaviors usually begin before the age of 15 and continue into adult life.
3. May be hospitalized for injuries.

B. Assessment findings
   1. Manipulative behavior, may try to obtain special privileges, play one staff member against another
   2. Lack of shame or guilt for behaviors
   3. Insincerity and lying
   4. Impulsive behavior and poor judgment
C. Nursing interventions
   1. Provide model for mature, appropriate behavior.
   2. Observe strict limit-setting by all staff.
   3. Monitor own responses to client.
   4. Demonstrate concern, interest in client.
   5. Reinforce positive behaviors (socialization, conforming to limits).
   6. Avoid power struggles.

REVIEW QUESTIONS

1. A 6-year-old has been diagnosed with enuresis after tests revealed no organic cause of bed wetting. The child's mother is upset and blames the problem on his father. "It's all his father's fault!" Your initial response is
   1. "Why do you say that?"
   2. "It's usually nobody's fault."
   3. "You seem really upset by this."
   4. "Why are you blaming his father?"

2. A 17-year-old is admitted with anorexia nervosa. You have been assigned to sit with her while she eats her dinner. The client says to you, "My primary nurse trusts me. I don't see why you don't." Your best response is
   1. "I do trust you, but I was assigned to be with you."
   2. "It sounds as if you are manipulating me."
   3. "OK. When I return, you should have eaten everything."
   4. "Who is your primary nurse?"

3. A 15-year-old is hospitalized for the treatment of anorexia nervosa. She is 64 inches tall and weighs 100 pounds. The primary objective in the treatment of the hospitalized anorexic client is to
   1. decrease the client's anxiety.
   2. increase insight into the disorder.
   3. help the mother to relinquish control.
   4. get the client to eat and gain weight.

4. A 15-year-old is hospitalized for treatment of anorexia nervosa. While admitting the client, the nurse discovers a bottle of pills that she calls

antacids. She takes them because her stomach hurts. The nurse's best initial response is

1. "Tell me more about your stomach pain."

2. "These do not look like antacids. I need to get an order for you to have them."

3. "Tell me more about your drug use."

4. "Some girls take pills to help them lose weight."

5. A nursing intervention based on the behavior modification model of treatment for anorexia would be

   1. role playing the client's interactions with her parents.

   2. encouraging the client to vent her feelings through exercise.

   3. providing a high-calorie, high-protein diet with between-meal snacks.

   4. restricting the client's privileges until she gains 3 pounds.

6. A 74-year-old was recently admitted to a nursing home because of confusion, disorientation, and negativistic behavior. Her family states that she is in good health. The woman asks you, "Where am I?" The best response for the nurse to make is

   1. "Don't worry. You're safe here."

   2. "Where do you think you are?"

   3. "What did your family tell you?"

   4. "You're at the community nursing home."

7. Which of the following would be an appropriate strategy in reorienting a confused client to where her room is?

   1. Place pictures of her family on the bedside stand.

   2. Put her name in large letters on her forehead.

   3. Remind the client where her room is.

   4. Let the other residents know where the client's room is.

8. A 74-year-old was recently admitted to a nursing home because of confusion, disorientation, and negativistic behavior. Which activity would you engage the client in at the nursing home?

   1. Reminiscence groups.

   2. Sing-alongs.

   3. Discussion groups.

   4. Exercise class.

9. A 78-year-old was recently admitted to a nursing home because of confusion, disorientation, and negativistic behavior. She has had difficulty

sleeping since admission. Which of the following would be the best intervention?

1. Provide her with a glass of warm milk.
2. Ask the physician for a mild sedative.
3. Do not allow her to take naps during the day.
4. Ask her family what they prefer.

10. A 46-year-old is on the verge of losing his job because of a drinking problem. He voluntarily enters an alcohol detoxification program. The most important information for him to accurately relate to the staff when admitted for detoxification is the amount, type, and

1. time substances were taken over the past 24 hours.
2. frequency of substances taken over the past week.
3. frequency of substances taken over the past 2 weeks.
4. frequency of substances taken over the past month.

11. A characteristic common to most substance abusers is difficulty in effectively

1. coping with stress and anxiety.
2. interacting socially.
3. performing in work-related settings.
4. setting limits.

12. Signs and symptoms that a client is developing impending alcohol withdrawal delirium include diaphoresis, tremors,

1. bradycardia, and hypertension.
2. bradycardia, and hypotension.
3. tachycardia, and hypertension.
4. tachycardia, and hypotension.

13. The most widely accepted treatment modality for substance abuse is

1. individual therapy with a psychodynamically oriented therapist.
2. individual therapy with a systems-oriented therapist.
3. group therapy with others with personality disorders.
4. group therapy with other substance abusers.

14. A 23-year-old man was voluntarily admitted to the inpatient unit with a diagnosis of paranoid schizophrenia. As the nurse approaches the client, he says, "If you come any closer, I'll die." This is an example of

1. hallucination.
2. delusion.

3. illusion.

4. idea of reference.

15. The nurse is approaching an adult client who is admitted with a diagnosis of paranoid schizophrenia. As the nurse approaches the client, he says, "If you come any closer, I'll die."The best response for the nurse to make to this behavior is

   1. "How can I hurt you?"

   2. "I'm the nurse."

   3. "Tell me more about this."

   4. "That's a silly thing to say."

16. A young man admitted with a diagnosis of paranoid schizophrenia is pacing the halls and is agitated. The nurse hears him saying, "I have to get away from those doctors! They are trying to commit me to the state hospital!" The nurse's continued assessment should include

   1. clarifying information with the doctor.

   2. observing the client for rising anxiety.

   3. reviewing history of involuntary commitment.

   4. checking dosage of prescribed medication.

17. When communicating with a paranoid client, the main principle is to

   1. use logic and be persistent.

   2. provide an anxiety-free environment.

   3. express doubt and do not argue.

   4. encourage ventilation of anger.

18. An appropriate activity for the nurse to recommend for a client who is extremely agitated is

   1. competitive sports.

   2. Bingo.

   3. Trivial Pursuit.

   4. daily walks.

19. The nurse knows that the major factor that distinguishes a bipolar from a unipolar disorder is the

   1. higher incidence in women.

   2. severity of the depression.

   3. genetic etiology.

   4. presence of mania.

20. A 34-year-old is hospitalized with bipolar disorder. At 2 A.M. the nurse finds him phoning friends all across the country to discuss his new plan for eradicating world hunger. His excited explanations are keeping the entire unit awake, but he won't quiet down. The nurse caring for him knows the drug most likely to be prescribed for this client is

    1. a tricyclic antidepressant.
    2. an MAO-inhibitor antidepressant.
    3. lithium carbonate (Eskalith).
    4. an antianxiety drug.

21. Supportive therapy for a client who is exhibiting manic behavior may include all of the following except

    1. psychoanalysis.
    2. cognitive therapy.
    3. interpersonal therapy.
    4. problem-solving therapy.

22. A 38-year-old was admitted to the psychiatric service after a failed suicide attempt by drug overdose. She had been in treatment with a clinical psychologist on a biweekly basis for 6 weeks. The client sought help when her husband informed her of his decision to leave her and the children after 19 years of marriage. Her suicide attempt was made after she and her husband had had a fierce argument about property settlement. Upon initial contact with the nurse, the client looked exhausted, affect was sad, movements and responses were slowed, and self-care impairments were evident. She is convinced that a blemish on her face is a melanoma that is invading her brain and eating away at the tissue. This client's disorder is best classified as

    1. bipolar disorder.
    2. depression with melancholia.
    3. dysthymic disorder.
    4. major depression.

23. An adult is admitted to the psychiatric service after a failed suicide attempt by drug overdose. She presents with a sad affect and moves and responds slowly. Which nursing diagnosis is of greatest priority at the time of her admission?

    1. Imbalanced in nutrition: less than body requirements.
    2. Ineffective coping.
    3. Risk for violence: self-directed.
    4. Bathing/hygiene self-care deficit.

24. An adult is admitted following a suicide attempt. She took sleeping pills. She has been receiving therapy for depression since her husband left her

after 23 years of marriage. Upon admission she looks very tired, has a sad affect, and moves slowly. In attempting to stabilize her activities of daily living in an optimally therapeutic way, she and the nurse would most likely plan to

1. allow her to catch up on lost sleep for the first 3 days of her hospitalization.

2. have her fully involved in all therapeutic activities.

3. have her husband visit for brief periods of time.

4. schedule balanced periods of rest and therapeutic activity.

25. The nurse suspects a client is denying his feelings of anxiety. When assessing this client, the nurse must be particularly alert to

1. restlessness.

2. tapping of the feet.

3. wringing of the hands.

4. his or her own anxiety level.

26. A 46-year-old is admitted to the hospital because her family is unable to manage her constant handwashing rituals. Her family reports she washes her hands at least 30 times each day. The nurse noticed the client's hands are reddened, scaly, and cracked. The main nursing goal is to

1. decrease the number of hand washings a day.

2. limit the number of hand washings.

3. provide good skin care.

4. eliminate the handwashing rituals.

27. An adult is admitted to the psychiatric hospital for handwashing rituals. The day after admission she is scheduled for lab tests. To ensure that the client is there on time, the nurse should

1. remind the client several times of her appointment.

2. limit the number of hand washings.

3. tell her it is her responsibility to be there on time.

4. provide ample time for her to complete her rituals.

28. An adult who is hospitalized with an obsessive-compulsive disorder washes her hands many times a day. Which of the following is an appropriate treatment for this client?

1. An unstructured schedule of activities.

2. A structured schedule of activities.

3. Intense counseling.

4. Negative reinforcement every time she performs the ritual.

29. A woman is admitted to the psychiatric hospital.She was found walking on a highway. She is unkempt and appears thin and dirty. The most thorough way to conduct a nursing assessment of her nutritional status is to

   1. observe her at mealtime.

   2. request a medical consult.

   3. explore her recent dietary intake.

   4. compare current weight with her usual

30. A 34-year-old is admitted to the psychiatric unit after she was brought to the hospital emergency department by the state police. She had been wandering on a major four-lane highway with no regard for her safety. On first contact with her, the nurse observes that her face and hands are very red and excoriated, her hair is matted and dirty, her clothing is dirty, and she is quite thin. According to the client, she had been living in a motel with a truck driver, whom she knew by first name only. They had been in the motel for a week, but the truck driver went back to work, and she has been alone for 3 days. She cannot specifically relate her activities for those 3 days. Once the assessment interview was over, she asked to be excused, went directly to her room, and washed her hands and face. Within a very short while, it became apparent to the nurse that the hand and face washing was quite repetitive and ritualistic and occupied a major portion of her time. However, she refused to bathe or wash her clothing. The nursing diagnosis that describes the most prominent difficulty that the client is experiencing is

   1. impaired skin integrity.

   2. disturbed thought processes.

   3. ineffective coping.

   4. social isolation.

31. An adult is admitted because of ritualistic behavior. She is also constipated and dehydrated. Which nursing intervention would the client be most likely to comply with?

   1. Drinking Ensure between meals.

   2. Drinking extra fluids with meals.

   3. Drinking 8 oz water every hour between meals.

   4. Drinking adequate amounts of fluid during the day.

32. An adult is admitted because of excessive hand and face washing rituals. The most effective way for the nurse to intervene with her hand and face washing is to

   1. allow her a certain amount of time each shift to engage in this behavior.

   2. interrupt the activity briefly and frequently.

   3. lock the door to her room and restrict access to the bathroom.

   4. tell her to stop each time she is observed doing it.

33. An adult was admitted for ritualistic behavior involving frequent hand and face washing. Upon admission she was also dehydrated and underweight. The nurse and the client will know that discharge planning is appropriate when the client

   1. regains her normal body weight.

   2. expresses a desire to leave the hospital.

   3. is able to start talking about her guilt and anxiety.

   4. limits her hand and face washing to a few times a day.

34. A young adult was admitted on a voluntary basis to psychiatric services. He had agreed to inpatient care as an alternative to a 30-day jail sentence for reckless driving, driving under the influence, and speeding. He has been under psychiatric care for three years, has a long history of petty crimes, and was able, with the help of his therapist, to convince the judge that a higher level of psychiatric care would be in everyone's best interest. Once on the unit, the client is difficult to manage because he is arrogant and manipulative. When a scheduled group therapy session is announced, he refuses to go and the nurse has to resort to pleading with him to attend. He uses other clients to his own ends and often pioneers causes that are disruptive to the milieu. The diagnostic title that best describes his behavior is

   1. antisocial personality disorder.

   2. borderline personality disorder.

   3. passive-aggressive personality disorder.

   4. passive-dependent personality disorder.

35. An adult is admitted to a psychiatric unit with a diagnosis of antisocial personality disorder. In planning care for the client it is important for the nurse to recognize that all of the following are likely to occur except

   1. staff and client agree when setting treatment goals.

   2. staff and client are in a constant struggle for control of the milieu.

   3. staff and client feel threatened by one another.

   4. staff and client use the same defense mechanisms when interacting.

36. Key interventions for a client with an antisocial personality disorder include all of the following except

   1. assisting him to identify and clarify his feelings.

   2. changing staff assigned to a client at his request.

3. making expectations about his behavior clear as well as consequences for same.

4. setting firm limits with clear consequences.

37. A 26-year-old man has been hospitalized with an antisocial personality disorder. He was admitted on a voluntary basis as an alternative to serving a jail sentence. At the time of discharge the nurse understands that the client is most likely to

1. be committed to another facility for a longer length of stay.

2. be committed to a virtuous and socially acceptable lifestyle.

3. discontinue treatment with the outpatient therapist.

4. revert to prehospitalization behaviors.

38. A 28-years old is admitted to the psychiatric unit under an involuntary petition after a perceived suicide attempt. The client cut the palmar aspect of her arm from the antecubital space to the hand. Immediately before this episode, she had flown across the country to return to her parents' home after her husband of one and a half years left her. Initially, she presented as very tearful and highly anxious. Her affect was more that of intense anger than of sadness. As the staff became more familiar with her, it became apparent that she had had many episodes of self-mutilation and would do so "so I can feel something." While she could appear quite intact most of the time, when stressed she would respond very impulsively, report hearing voices of a depreciative nature, and require a high level of observation. As the end of her hospitalization neared, she became increasingly angry, anxious, and hostile, saying, "You people (the staff) are useless. You can't help anyone get better. Look at me, I'm no better than when I came in." This client's symptoms can best be described as fitting which of the following diagnostic categories?

1. Antisocial personality disorder.

2. Borderline personality disorder.

3. Passive-aggressive personality disorder.

4. Passive-dependent personality disorder.

39. An adult is admitted to the psychiatric unit with a diagnosis of borderline personality disorder.All of the following components of a nursing history/ data base are extremely important to explore with this client except

1. ego-strength assessment.

2. social history.

3. cognitive aspect of mental status exam.

4. past psychiatric treatment history.

40. An adult was admitted to the psychiatric unit after cutting herself on the forearm. She has numerous scars which are from prior self-mutilation. Should the client attempt self-mutilation while in the hospital, the plan for the nurse to implement is

   1. focus on the how, when, and where of the injury.

   2. care for the injury and explore the client's activities and feelings immediately before the episode.

   3. care for the injury and leave the client alone for a while to let her settle down.

   4. care for the injury and seclude, and possibly restrain, the client to prevent further injury.

41. A young woman was admitted with a borderline personality disorder following an episode of self-mutilation. Her husband recently left her. She seems angry much of the time. She reports that she has injured herself in the past so she could feel something. In evaluating her as she nears discharge, the nurse would identify the major issues during this hospitalization to be all of the following except

   1. cognition.

   2. identity.

   3. dealing with anger.

   4. separation/individuation.

42. while collecting data about a 7-year-old boy, the school nurse learned that he has minimal verbal skills and expresses his needs by acting out behaviors. The communication capabilities of this boy indicate which of the following levels of mental retardation?

   1. Mild.

   2. Moderate.

   3. Severe.

   4. Profound.

43. The nursing care for a 4-year-old boy with severe autistic disorder is most likely to include

   1. psychotropic medications.

   2. social skills training.

   3. play therapy.

   4. group therapy.

44. The nurse makes the following assessment of a 14-year-old gymnast: underweight, hair loss, yellowish skin, facial lanugo, and peripheral edema. These findings are suggestive of which of the following disorders?

1. Anorexia nervosa.

2. Bulimia nervosa.

3. Acquired immunodeficiency.

4. Ulcerative colitis.

45. A 15-year-old gymnast presents in the eating disorders clinic severely emaciated, with sallow skin color, 20% body weight loss, amenorrhea for the past 12 months, and facial lanugo. Based on these findings, which one of the following nursing diagnoses would be most appropriate for the nurse to make?

1. Impaired nutrition: less than body requirements.

2. Impaired tissue integrity.

3. Ineffective individual coping.

4. Deficient knowledge, nutritional.

46. Which observation of the client with anorexia indicates the client is improving?

1. The client eats meals in the dining room.

2. The client gains 1 pound per week.

3. The client attends group therapy sessions.

4. The client has a more realistic self-concept.

47. A client with severe Alzheimer's disease has violent outbursts, wanders, and is incontinent.He can no longer identify familiar people or objects. In developing the nursing care plan, the nurse would give highest priority to which nursing diagnosis?

1. High risk for injury.

2. Impaired verbal communication.

3. Self-care deficits.

4. Altered pattern of urinary elimination: incontinence.

48. A client with Alzheimer's disease has a self-care deficit related to his cognitive impairment. He has difficulty dressing himself. The best action for the nurse to take is to

1. have the client wear hospital gowns.

2. explain to the client why he should dress himself.

3. give the client step-by-step instructions for dressing himself.

4. allow enough time for the client to dress himself.

49. The family of a client with Alzheimer's disease indicates to the nurse an understanding of the prognosis when they say,

1. "Does another hospital have a better treatment?"

2. "Will a change in diet help his memory?"

3.   "Won't his new medicine cure him?"

4.   "What supports are available for the long haul?"

50. A 75-year-old man was brought to the emergency room confused, incoherent, and agitated after painting his lawn furniture earlier in the day. He has no current history of illness. Which one of the following interpretations would be appropriate for the nurse to make about his condition?

1.   Depression related to aging.

2.   Dementia related to organic illness.

3.   Delirium related to toxin exposure.

4.   Distress related to unaccomplished tasks.

51. A student with a history of barbiturate addiction is brought to the infirmary with suspected overdose. Which of the following assessments is the nurse likely to make?

1.   Watery eyes, slow and shallow breathing, clammy skin.

2.   Dilated pupils, shallow respirations, weak and rapid pulse.

3.   Constricted pupils, respirations depressed, nausea.

4.   Responsive pupils, increased respirations, increased pulse and blood pressure.

52. A 16-year-old girl is admitted to a detoxification unit with a history of cocaine abuse. Her pupils are dilated and she complains of nausea and feeling cold. She states that she is not addicted, but uses cocaine occasionally with friends. Which one of the following nursing diagnoses is appropriate for the nurse to make?

1.   Impaired verbal communication related to substance use as evidenced by giving untrue information.

2.   Altered growth and development related to substance use as evidenced by age of client.

3.   Perceptual alteration related to substance use as evidenced by distortion of reality.

4.   Ineffective denial related to substance use as evidenced in refusal to admit problem.

53. The nursing care plan for a client in early alcohol withdrawal is most likely to include

1.   using physical restraints.

2.   providing environmental stimulation.

3.   taking pulse and blood pressure.

4.   administering antipsychotic medications.

54. A client in a detox program is being manipulative by trying to split staff and ingratiating himself with certain clients. The best response of the nurse to being told he or she is the "best" staff member on the unit is to

    1. thank the client for the compliment.

    2. identify the client's manipulative behavior.

    3. ignore the client's comment.

    4. ask the client why he feels that way.

55. In developing a teaching plan for adolescents on the topic of cocaine abuse, the nurse would highlight which of the following?

    1. Cocaine is a naturally occurring depressant.

    2. Cocaine's physical effects differ according to the method of ingestion.

    3. The body's peak reaction occurs 30 minutes after it is taken.

    4. Taking cocaine by injection is particularly dangerous to the cardiovascular system.

56. A 14-year-old male client is admitted to the emergency room after ingesting a high dose of PCP and subsequently injuring himself in a fall. An effective action for the nurse to take is to

    1. attempt to talk the client down.

    2. withhold fluids.

    3. place the client in a quiet, dimly lit room.

    4. administer a prn phenothiazine.

57. The nurse on a medical unit smells alcohol and notices that the relief nurse's words are slurred and she is giggling inappropriately. The best initial action for the nurse to take is to

    1. double assign the nurse's clients.

    2. ask the relief nurse if she has been drinking.

    3. report the nurse to the licensing board.

    4. refer the nurse to an employee assistance program.

58. A staff nurse observes another nurse diverting meperidine (Demerol) ordered for a client and injecting it into herself. The nurse denies that she has done anything wrong and pleads with her colleague to remain quiet. What is the best action for the staff nurse?

    1. Agree to remain quiet if the nurse promises to enter treatment.

    2. Notify the nurse manager/supervisor.

    3. Notify a family member of the nurse.

    4. Send the nurse home without saying anything.

59. The nurse evaluates that an adult may be ready for discharge from the substance abuse unit when she says,

   1. "I'll take my Antabuse when I need it."

   2. "I can't wait to hang out with my old buddies."

   3. "I'll drink in moderation and only on the weekend."

   4. "Attending daily AA meetings will help me not drink again."

60. Which of the following assessment findings would the nurse observe in a client with schizophrenia?

   1. Associative looseness, affect disturbance, ambivalence, autistic thinking.

   2. Euphoria, distractibility, dramatic mannerisms, energetic.

   3. Argumentative, anhedonia, poor judgment, manipulative.

   4. Psychomotor retardation, intense sadness, loss of energy, suicidal.

61. A client with a diagnosis of paranoid schizophrenia reports to the nurse that he hears a voice that says, "Don't take those poisoned pills from that nurse!" Which one of the following nursing diagnoses would it be appropriate for the nurse to make regarding this statement?

   1. Disturbed sensory perceptual: auditory, related to anxiety as evidenced by auditory hallucination.

   2. Disturbed thought processes related to anxiety as evidenced by delusions of persecution.

   3. Defensive coping related to impaired reality testing as evidenced by paranoid ideation.

   4. Impaired verbal communication related to disturbances in form of thinking as evidenced by use of symbolic references.

62. An adult is admitted with a diagnosis of catatonic schizophrenia, excited phase. She shouts and paces continuously and seems to be responding to internal stimuli. A realistic short-term goal for the nurse to formulate is

   1. the client will groom self daily.

   2. the client will maintain adequate nutrition.

   3. the client will sleep 8 hours per night.

   4. the client will attend unit social activities.

63. A client with schizophrenia stops talking mid sentence and tilts her head to one side. The nurse suspects that the client is experiencing auditory hallucinations. The best initial action is for the nurse to

   1. ask the client what she is experiencing

   2. change the topic of conversation.

3. explain that hallucinations are not real.

4. deny that she hears anything.

64. In teaching a client for whom clozapine (Clozaril) has been prescribed, the nurse would include which of the following?

1. The drug will be given every four weeks by intramuscular injection.

2. The drug will probably cause weight reduction.

3. There is a high incidence of extrapyramidal side effects.

4. The signs and symptoms of blood dyscrasia.

65. An adult is to go on a 3-day pass and has his maintenance supply of chlorpromazine (Thorazine). Which statement indicates to the nurse that he understands instructions regarding his medication?

1. "I'll take my pills when I hear those voices."

2. "I'll drink beer but no wine while I'm away."

3. "I'll cover up when I go to the beach."

4. "I'll stop taking it if my mouth stays dry."

66. Which of the following behaviors indicates to the nurse that the client's antipsychotic medication is having a desired effect?

1. The client states that her "voices" are not as threatening.

2. The client reports having inner feelings of restlessness.

3. The client sleeps all day.

4. The client reports muscular stiffening in her face and arms.

67. A client taking trifluoperazine (Stelazine) exhibits severe extrapyramidal symptoms, a temperature of 105°F, and diaphoresis. The nurse suspects neuroleptic malignant syndrome.The best action of the nurse is to

1. administer an antiparkinsonism medication.

2. stop the neuroleptic medication.

3. withhold fluids.

4. administer an antianxiety medication.

68. A client with paranoid schizophrenia has a delusion of persecution. He tells the nurse, "The CIA is out to get me. They're spying on me." The nurse's best initial response is,

1. "I don't want to hurt you."

2. "How would they spy on you here?"

3. "Tell me how they're trying to get you."

4. "I know the CIA wouldn't want to hurt you."

69. Which of the following statements indicates to the nurse that a client with obsessive-compulsive disorder has developed insight into her problem?

    1. "I realize that the dangers are more in my mind."
    2. "I don't hear the voices anymore."
    3. "I check on my family 12 times every day."
    4. "I slept 8 hours last night."

70. An adult is brought to the emergency room after he attempted to walk across the roof of a building in an attempt to "fly like a jet plane." In addition to impulsiveness, which of the behaviors identified below would the nurse assess in a client diagnosed as bipolar, manic type?

    1. Hallucinations and delusions.
    2. Euphoria and increased motor activity.
    3. Paranoia and ideas of reference.
    4. Splitting and manipulation.

71. During the focused assessment of a client with major depression, the nurse may ask which of the following questions?

    1. "You seem to have a lot of energy; when did you last have 6 or more hours of sleep?"
    2. "You seem to be angry with your family now; when was it that you last got along?"
    3. "Have you had any thoughts of harming yourself?"
    4. "You seem to be listening to something. Could you tell me about it?"

72. Which of the following nursing diagnoses would be most appropriate for a client who is diagnosed as bipolar I disorder, single manic episode and is intrusive, argumentative, and severely critical of peers?

    1. Impaired social interaction related to narcissistic behavior as evidenced by inability to sustain relationships.
    2. Risk for injury related to extreme hyperactivity as evidenced by increased agitation and lack of control over behavior.
    3. Social isolation related to feelings of inadequacy in social interaction as evidence by problematic interaction with others.
    4. Defensive coping related to social learning patterns as evidenced by difficulty interacting with others.

73. An adult is in an acute manic phase of bipolar disorder. He talks and paces incessantly, frequently shouting and threatening other clients. The nurse expects the client's care plan to include which of the following?

1. Monitor blood lithium levels.

2. Monitor client during phototherapy.

3. Monitor client after electroconvulsive therapy.

4. Teach client to avoid foods with tyramine.

74. The nurse is preparing to administer lithium (Eskalith) to a client with bipolar disorder. The client complains of nausea and muscle weakness, and his speech is slurred. His lithium level is 1.6 mEq/L. The best action for the nurse to take is to

1. chart the client's symptoms after giving the lithium.

2. explain that these are common side-effects.

3. withhold the client's lithium.

4. administer a prn antiparkinsonism drug.

75. Which of the following behaviors indicates to the nurse that the client understands her teaching related to lithium treatment? The client

1. takes her lithium 1 hour after meals.

2. states she will stop taking her lithium when her mania subsides.

3. goes on a low salt diet to counter weight gain.

4. states she will withhold her lithium if she experiences diarrhea, vomiting, and diaphoresis.

76. An adult is recovering from a severe depression. Which of the following behaviors alerts the nurse to a risk for suicide?

1. The client sleeps most of the day.

2. The client has a plan to kill herself.

3. The client loses 5 pounds.

4. The client does not attend unit activities.

77. A man has been severely depressed for 2 weeks. He had mentioned "ending it all" prior to admission. Which of the following questions should the nurse ask during the prescreen assessment?

1. "How long have you thought about harming yourself?"

2. "What is it that makes you think about harming yourself?"

3. "How has your concentration been?"

4. "What specifically have you thought about doing to harm yourself?"

78. A 19-year-old recently broke off her 1-year engagement. Her mother states, "She does nothing but cry and sit and stare into space. I can't get her to eat or anything!" She feels she can't go on without her boyfriend. The nurse should make which priority nursing diagnosis?

1. Impaired nutrition: less than body requirements.
2. Dysfunctional grieving.
3. Risk for self-directed violence.
4. Social isolation.

79. An adult is admitted for treatment of a major depression. She is withdrawn, appears disheveled, and states, "No one could ever love me." The nurse can expect the client to be placed on

1. antiparkinsonism medication.
2. suicide precautions.
3. a low-salt diet.
4. phototherapy.

80. A man's wife complains that her husband's depression isn't any better after 1 week on amitriptyline (Elavil). The nurse's best response is to

1. tell her she will contact the physician.
2. question the wife about what response she expects.
3. explain that it may take 1 to 3 weeks to see any improvement.
4. suggest that the client change antidepressants.

81. Which of the following behaviors indicates to the nurse that a client's major depression is improving? The client

1. displays a blunted affect.
2. has lost an additional 2 pounds.
3. states one "good" thing about himself.
4. sleeps about 16 hours per day.

82. An adult is hospitalized for treatment of obsessive-compulsive disorder (OCD). The nurse recognizes which of the following as an indication that the client's sertraline (Zoloft) is having the desired effect?

1. The client experiences nervousness and drowsiness.
2. The client's delusions are less entrenched.
3. The client engages in fewer rituals.
4. The client sleeps 4 hours per night.

83. A client with major depression is scheduled for electroconvulsive therapy (ECT) tomorrow. The nurse would plan for which of the following activities?

1. Force fluids 6 to 8 hours before treatment.
2. Administer succinylcholine (Inestine, Anectine) during pretreatment care.
3. Encourage the client's spouse to accompany him.
4. Reorient the client frequently during posttreatment care.

84. A severely depressed client received ECT this morning. Which of the findings listed below would the nurse *least* expect to assess posttreatment?

    1. Headache.
    2. Memory loss.
    3. Paralytic ileus.
    4. Disorientation.

85. A client for whom Nardil was prescribed for depression is brought to the ER with severe occipital headaches after eating pepperoni pizza for lunch. Which of the following interpretations is it important for the nurse to make regarding these findings?

    1. Allergic reaction related to ingestion of processed food.
    2. Hypertensive crisis related to drug and food reaction.
    3. Panic anxiety related to unresolved issues.
    4. Conversion disorder related to uncontrolled anxiety.

86. The nurse understands that the major difference between neurotic disorders and psychotic disorders is that in psychotic disorders the clients

    1. are aware that their behaviors are maladaptive.
    2. are aware they are experiencing distress.
    3. experience no loss of contact with reality.
    4. exhibit a flight from reality.

87. The nurse realizes that a client taking buspirone hydrochloride (BuSpar) needs additional medication teaching when he says,

    1. "I'll take my drugs as soon as I feel anxious."
    2. "I won't drink any alcohol."
    3. "I'll report any troubles with my heart or seeing."
    4. "I'll have my blood checked every month."

88. In teaching a client about her new antianxiety medication, alprazolam (Xanax), the nurse should include which of the following?

    1. Caution the client to avoid foods with tyramine.
    2. Caution the client not to drink alcoholic beverages.
    3. Instruct the client to take the Xanax 1 hour after meals.
    4. Instruct the client to double up a dose if she forgets to take her medication.

89. A client experiencing thanataphobia is afraid to leave her aging, ailing husband alone for any reason. She has not left her husband alone since her mother and sister died 4 years ago. Which of the following statements

would be appropriate for the nurse to make during the initial assessment of this client?

1. "Are you afraid that your husband might die while you are away from him?"

2. "There must be someone you are able to trust to stay with your husband."

3. "Don't you have children who are willing to stay with your husband when you need to be away?"

4. "It must be very confining to have constantly attended to your husband for so long."

90. A newly admitted client is fearful of elevators. She needs to take one in 10 minutes to attend therapy on the 10th floor. Which of the following actions would be best for the nurse to take?

1. Explain to her that she needs to attend therapy.

2. Have another client go with her.

3. Accompany her to the 10th floor.

4. Explore with her why she is afraid of elevators.

91. A man, with a family of five, was recently laid off and now has financial concerns. He is experiencing muscle tension, breathlessness, and sleep disturbances. Which one of the following nursing diagnoses would be appropriate for the nurse to make regarding his condition?

1. Post-trauma response related to loss of economic support as evidenced by job loss.

2. Parental role conflict related to perceived inability to meet his family's economic and physical needs as evidenced by job loss.

3. Ineffective individual coping related to recent unemployment as evidenced by physical manifestations.

4. Powerlessness related to inability to deal with anxiety as evidenced by physical manifestations.

92. A woman appears to be having a panic attack during group therapy. She is agitated, pacing rapidly, and not responding to verbal stimuli. The best initial nursing intervention is to

1. remove her from the group.

2. encourage her to express her feelings.

3. facilitate her recognizing her anxiety.

4. ignore her.

93. The nurse is assessing a client who presents with OCD. In addition to gathering information about the client's anxiety and rituals, the nurse should assess for which of the following?

1. Handwringing and foot-tapping behaviors.
2. Use of abusive substances and gambling.
3. Tics, stuttering, or other unusual speech patterns.
4. Diaphoresis and rapid breathing.

94. Which of the following statements by a client with delusions indicates to the nurse that the client is improving?
   1. "I don't feel those crawling bugs anymore."
   2. "I won't talk about my crazy thoughts at work."
   3. "I feel less jumpy inside."
   4. "I must check my room for bugs."

95. During the assessment phase of the nurse-client interaction, which of the following statements made by the client is suggestive of post-traumatic stress disorder?
   1. "My dad had trouble swallowing before he died and I always feel as if I have a lump in my throat."
   2. "After I contracted meningitis on vacation last summer, I can't control this horrible thought that all people who work in park restaurants are dirty."
   3. "I continue to have the same dream over and over again. At least once a month."
   4. "I had another horrible nightmare last night and went through the same trauma and anxiety all over again."

96. A client with OCD has an elaborate handwashing and touching ritual that interferes with her activities of daily living. She misses meals and therapy sessions. The nurse recognizes that an effective strategy to limit her ritual is to
   1. teach thought stopping techniques.
   2. prevent the ritualistic behavior.
   3. use adjunctive therapies for distraction.
   4. facilitate her insight regarding the need for the ritual.

97. A client with an OCD has checking rituals and thoughts that her family will be harmed. Which of the following indicates to the nurse that the client is improving? The client
   1. obsesses about her family's health.
   2. adheres to the unit schedule.
   3. loses 2 pounds in 1 week.
   4. awakens 8 times during the night.

98. A 4-year-old girl who is a victim of a bomb blast that demolished the building which housed her daycare constantly builds block houses and blows them up. She also has nightmares frequently. Which one of the following diagnoses is appropriate for the nurse to make regarding this child?

1. Post-trauma response related to terrorist attack as evidenced by destructive behaviors and sleep disturbances.

2. Explosive disorder related to dysfunctional personality as evidenced by destructive behaviors.

3. Sleep disturbance related to emotional trauma as evidenced by nightmares.

4. Ineffective individual coping related to internal stressors as evidenced by destructive behaviors and nightmares.

99. The nurse recognizes that the client with post-traumatic stress disorder (PTSD) is improving when he

1. states he feels "numb" most of the time.

2. drinks alcohol to cope with his feelings.

3. talks about a benefit of the traumatic experience.

4. attends weekly group therapy.

100. A young woman is found wandering on campus after a fraternity party. She is disheveled and does not know who she is. She has no recollection of the evening. At the student health service she is diagnosed with dissociative amnesia subsequent to a rape. The most appropriate nursing diagnosis for the nurse to formulate is

1. ineffective individual coping.

2. personal identity disturbance.

3. anxiety related to alteration in memory.

4. risk for violence, self-directed.

101. The nurse finds, during the initial assessment of the star player on the basketball team, that he is not concerned about the sudden paralysis of his "shooting arm." This behavior is known as

1. secondary gain.

2. la belle indifference.

3. malingering.

4. hypochondriasis.

102. A man's family brought him into the hospital because of his many somatic complaints. He has been seen by many medical specialists in the past without discovery of organic pathology. The nurse assesses that the client is probably experiencing which of the following problems?

1. Conversion disorder.
2. Body dysmorphic disorder.
3. Malingering.
4. Hypochondriasis.

103. An adult is hospitalized for treatment of a conversion disorder. She complained of paralysis of her right side after her husband threatened to leave her and their children. She seems unconcerned about her paralysis. An appropriate long-term goal for the nurse to formulate is that the client will

1. cope effectively with stress without using conversion.
2. identify stressors.
3. express feelings about the conflict.
4. develop an increased sense of relatedness to others.

104. An adult has hypochondriasis—believing he is dying of stomach cancer despite repeated and extensive diagnostic testing that has all been negative. He has become reclusive and is preoccupied with his physical complaints. The nurse would include which of the following in the nursing care plan? The client will

1. focus on the signs and symptoms of stomach cancer.
2. attend a support group for persons with cancer.
3. complete a contract to attend social and diversional activities daily.
4. receive secondary gain from his physical symptoms.

105. A man is brought into the police station after he ran toward a boy who resembled his son. At the police station he was unable to recall any personal information. The prescreening nurse inferred that the man has which one of the following dissociative disorders?

1. Amnesia.
2. Fugue.
3. Personality disorder.
4. Stress disorder.

106. Which of the behaviors listed below would assist the nurse in establishing the diagnosis of borderline personality disorder?

1. Impulsivity.
2. Hallucinations.
3. Self-mutilation.
4. Narcissism.

107. A woman is admitted to the unit with a diagnosis of borderline personality disorder. She has angry outbursts and is impulsive and

manipulative. She has lacerations on her arm from self-mutilation. The priority nursing diagnosis for the nurse to formulate is

1. ineffective individual coping.

2. disturbed body image.

3. disturbed personal identity.

4. risk for violence to self.

108. A client with borderline personality disorder tells the nurse she hates her doctor because he denied her a pass because she returned "high" from her last pass. The best nursing action for the nurse is to

1. ask the client why she is feeling so angry.

2. suggest that the client bring it up in community meeting.

3. offer to contact the doctor and discuss the situation.

4. set limits and point out that the denial is a consequence of her inappropriate behavior.

109. The nurse would formulate which of the following outcome criteria for a client with borderline personality disorder? The client

1. displays anger frequently.

2. acts out her neediness.

3. experiences troubling thoughts without self-mutilation.

4. idolizes her nurse.

110. A client with antisocial personality disorder is charming, seductive, and highly manipulative.He has a history of multiple jobs and marriages, which have all failed, and problems with the law. Which of the following is an appropriate short-term goal for the nurse to formulate in relation to a nursing diagnosis of ineffective individual coping? The client will

1. avoid situations that provoke aggressive acts.

2. adhere to unit rules.

3. assume a leadership role in unit governance.

4. acknowledge manipulative behaviors pointed out by staff.

111. Which of the following indicates to the nurse that a client with antisocial personality disorder is improving? The client

1. compliments the nurse for her outstanding job on the unit.

2. tests the limits on his behavior.

3. acknowledges some manipulative behavior.

4. sleeps 8 hours per night.

ANSWERS AND RATIONALES

1. **3.** Upon hearing her son's diagnosis, the mother is experiencing emotional turmoil and projecting blame. Acknowledging her feelings would build further trust and encourage her to discuss her thoughts and feelings.

2. **2.** Clients diagnosed with eating disorders usually have difficulty establishing trust. Confronting the client's manipulation assists her in dealing with this maladaptive behavior.

3. **4.** Because the anorexic client is experiencing starvation, her well-being is dependent on establishing an adequate nutritional state. Eating and gaining weight are the primary goals of hospitalization.

4. **1.** While there might be some concern that the client is abusing drugs and possibly using them to induce further weight loss, the primary concern is that the client is experiencing abdominal pain. This may be a clue to an impending medical crisis needing further assessment.

5. **4.** Behavior modification involves creating positive and negative consequences for desirable and undesirable behavior. The benefit of gaining weight is adding privileges.

6. **4.** Responding factually helps to orient the client.

7. **3.** The nurse should be someone the client can turn to for guidance.

8. **4.** Providing the client with structured activities will allow her to release tension. Exercises also help older people with balance and mobility and reduce falls.

9. **4.** Including the family in the plan of care ensures a more effective plan.

10. **1.** Although a complete substance abuse history is necessary eventually, on admission the most important information is the type and amount of substances taken by the client in the past 24 hours.

11. **1.** While a substance abuser has difficulty in all areas listed, problems handling stress and anxiety underlie all the others.

12. **3.** Delirium tremens is characterized by increased blood pressure, pulse, and respirations, and an increase in psychomotor activity.

13. **4.** Group therapy with other substance abusers is the most highly prescribed therapy. It is the model for Alcoholics Anonymous, the most effective treatment group.

14. **2.** A delusion is a fixed false belief.

15. **2.** The nurse needs to present reality to the client and not encourage the delusion.

16. 2. Assessing increasing signs of anxiety and agitation gives clues to the client's ability to maintain control and suggests further nursing interventions to protect the client and others.

17. 3. Paranoid clients develop a delusional system to defend against anxiety. Arguing with the client would increase his anxiety.

18. 4. Daily walks provide time for the nurse to develop trust. Walking allows expenditure of energy without increasing paranoia.

19. 4. Both unipolar and bipolar disorders include episodes of depression. The diagnosis of bipolar disorder is given to persons who also experience manic episodes.

20. 3. A drug frequently used to treat manic clients is lithium carbonate (Eskalith).

21. 1. Psychoanalysis is an in-depth, insight-oriented psychotherapy, not appropriate in treatment of bipolar disorders.

22. 4. The client shows many signs of classic depression as evidenced by psychomotor retardation, impairment of self-care, inability to sleep, a suicide attempt, and somatic delusion.

23. 3. The priority at this time is maintenance of client safety. This client is at particular risk for self-directed violence because of her recent failed suicide attempt and her obsession with what she perceives to be her impending death.

24. 4. Even though the client is probably exhausted, the most therapeutic plan would allow for both rest and activity.

25. 4. Clients who are unaware of or denying their feelings of anxiety are less likely to exhibit overt behavioral symptoms. The nurse should rely on the empathic, contagious communication of anxiety from client to nurse.

26. 1. Obsessive-compulsive behavior represents displacement of anxiety. A concrete measurable goal is to decrease the number of handwashings.

27. 4. Providing ample time for the client to complete her handwashing rituals will lessen her anxiety.

28. 2. Planning a structured schedule of activities provides the client with ways other than handwashing to reduce anxiety.

29. 4. Current weight as it relates to usual weight is the best determinant of nutritional status and weight change when the client is unable to be specific about recent activities and eating habits.

30. 3. Ineffective individual coping encompasses all of the other nursing diagnoses. This area will be the primary focus of nursing interventions, and positive changes in the client's ability to cope will be the criteria for discharge readiness.

31. 3. Building the intake of a specified amount of liquid into a daily schedule of activities is very consistent with the obsessive-compulsive client's need to control as many aspects of her life as possible.

32. 1. Allowing the client a certain amount of time to engage in the activity alleviates some of the client's anxiety.

33. 4. The major issue is control of behavior and thoughts. When the client is able to control her compulsive behavior, i.e., limit her hand and face washing to a few times a day, she will then be able to resume normal activities of daily living.

34. 1. A long history of petty crimes, a high level of manipulative behavior, use of other clients to his own end, and fostering behavior that is disruptive to the milieu are all signs of the diagnosis of antisocial personality disorder.

35. 1. The staff and client will most likely disagree when setting treatment goals.

36. 2. The client will compare and attempt to "split" staff, so it is very important to keep staff assignments as consistent as possible.

37. 4. People who have this type of personality disorder typically seek psychiatric care as a lesser of two evils. In this case in-hospital care is preferable to jail. The chances of this client making any great change in his lifestyle as a result of short-term hospitalization are slim. The client will likely be committed to another facility when he is again arrested for deviant behavior.

38. 2. The clustering of self-mutilation, impulsivity, transient psychosis, intense anger, and feeling empty is most typically found in borderline personality disorder.

39. 3. The mental status exam is conducted when the nurse suspects a client is disoriented. The client with a borderline personality disorder has, for the most part, intact reality testing.

40. 2. A matter-of-fact approach to the injury with emphasis on the events leading to the episode of mutilation is the most therapeutic approach.

41. 1. Impairments involving cognition are most commonly found in psychoses.

42. 3. Individuals with severe mental retardation possess minimal verbal skills. They often communicate wants and needs by acting out behaviors.

43. 3. Play therapy would be most effective given his developmental level and autism. In autistic disorder, communication with others is severely impaired. Through one-to-one play therapy, the therapist may establish rapport through nonverbal play.

44. 1. Anorexia nervosa, usually occurring in individuals ages 13–22 years, is an eating disorder characterized by self-starvation, weight loss (25% below normal weight), disturbance in body image, and physiologic and metabolic changes.

45. 1. The assessment data and history of the client support the diagnosis of altered nutrition related to anorexia.

46. 2. Weight gain is the best indication that the client's anorexia is improving. A realistic expectation is for the client to gain 1 pound per week.

47. 1. Safety is of highest concern for this client. His wandering and memory loss pose hazards for accidents, falls, and injuries.

48. 3. The client may need step-by-step instructions so he can focus on small amounts of information. This allows him to perform at his optimal level. Clients with dementia may not remember how to dress themselves.

49. 4. This response indicates that the family is expecting to need support during the process of the client's increasing cognitive impairment.

50. 3. Delirium is a state of mental confusion and excitement. The mind wanders, speech is incoherent, and the client is often in a state of continual, aimless physical activity. The onset is rapid (hours to days). Paint is a toxin that could cause delirium.

51. 2. The effects of overdose of barbiturates are shallow respirations, cold and clammy skin, dilated pupils, weak and rapid pulse, coma, and possible death.

52. 4. Denial is the minimizing or disavowing of symptoms or a situation to the detriment of health.

53. 3. Pulse and blood pressure should be checked hourly for the first 8–12 hours after admission.They are usually elevated during withdrawal and the pulse is a good indication of progress through withdrawal. Elevation may indicate impending alcohol withdrawal delirium.

54. 2. A priority in intervening in manipulative behavior is to identify it and then set limits by stating expected behaviors.

55. 4. A total cardiac collapse may occur. Freebasing is the method that most often leads to myocardial infarction.

56. 3. Environmental stimuli need to be reduced for the client in PCP intoxication to reduce danger to self, paranoia, delusions, and hallucinations.These clients are sensitive to stimuli and quickly become combative and assaultive.

57. 2. There is usually a chain of command policy that begins with a direct discussion of the involved parties. If the relief nurse denies drinking, the nurse has a duty to intervene.

58. 2. The hospital's chain of command policy must be followed. The duty to intervene to protect patients from harm must be followed in light of the nurse's poor judgment, etc.

59. 4. Daily attendance at AA meetings is necessary for most discharged clients to remain sober and continue their rehabilitation.

60. 1. Eugen Bleuler's 4 As of schizophrenia are loosening of associations (L.O.A.), which are representative of thought disorders, disturbance in affect, ambivalence, and autistic thinking.

61. 1. Hallucinations are sensory experiences of perception without corresponding stimuli in the environment.

62. 2. It is important for the nurse to monitor dietary intake and weight so the person does not lose calories and fluids due to hyperactivity. "Finger foods" may need to be provided, e.g., sandwiches and fruit.

63. 1. The best initial action is to focus on the cues and elicit the client's description of her experience. It is important for the nurse to determine that she is hallucinating and the content. This is vital in relation to safety issues and command hallucinations.

64. 4. Symptoms of blood dyscrasias such as sore throat, fever, malaise, unusual bleeding need to be taught. Weekly white blood cell counts may be required.

65. 3. The client should avoid the sun or cover up and use sunscreen to protect himself from severe photosensitivity.

66. 1. A desired effect of the antipsychotics is to reduce the disturbing quality of hallucinations and delusions.

67. 2. The neuroleptic should be immediately discontinued. Medical treatment should be instituted because this is a potentially fatal syndrome.

68. 1. The nurse should first clarify her intent and then empathize with the underlying feeling.

69. 1. This statement indicates that the client has some insight into the underlying reason for her rituals.

70. 2. The client diagnosed as bipolar, manic exhibits behaviors of elation, euphoria, and is full of energy, which may lead to exhaustion.

71. 3. Clients with major depression are often suicidal. The first concern of assessment is the risk of suicide potential in the immediate future.

72. 2. The client who invades the space of others, creates arguments, and attacks others is at risk for injury by those in the environment.

73. 1. Lithium is the drug of choice for manic clients with an antimanic effectiveness of 78%. It reduces the intensity, duration, and frequency of manic and depressive episodes. Blood levels are monitored for therapeutic levels in the acute phase (1.0–1.5 mEq/L) and during maintenance.

74. **3.** The client is exhibiting symptoms and signs of lithium toxicity. Another blood level should be drawn and the dose evaluated.

75. **4.** These are early signs of lithium toxicity. The drug should be withheld and a lithium blood level drawn and evaluated to determine an appropriate dosage.

76. **2.** Having a suicide plan is a risk factor. The lethality needs to be assessed. When a depression is "lifting," the client may have the energy and resources to carry out a plan. Behavioral, somatic, and emotional cues may be overt or covert.

77. **4.** This question assists in determining suicidal intent and lethality.

78. **3.** The depressed client often feels hopeless and helpless with self-directed anger. Suicidal ideations are often expressed and warrant immediate intervention.

79. **2.** Maintaining safety for the client is a priority because she may have suicidal ideation and/or a plan.

80. **3.** The client may need to take Elavil 1 to 3 weeks before any improvement or a therapeutic effect is noticed.

81. **3.** This behavior may indicate an increase in self-esteem that accompanies an improvement in depression. A depressed person often cannot problem solve or acknowledge any positive aspects of their lives.

82. **3.** Zoloft is a selective serotonin reuptake inhibitor (SSRI) that is effective in treating clients with obsessive-compulsive disorder. Using fewer rituals would indicate an improvement.

83. **4.** Common side effects of bilateral treatment include confusion, disorientation, and short-term memory loss. The nurse should provide frequent orientation statements that are brief, distinct, and simple.

84. **3.** ECT is treated as an operative procedure; however, paralytic ileus (intestinal obstruction, especially failure of peristalsis) frequently accompany peritonitis and usually result from disturbances in the bowel.

85. **2.** Severe occipital and/or temporal pounding headaches, manifestations of hypertensive crisis, occur when processed meats are eaten by individuals currently taking nardil (MAOI).

86. **4.** In psychotic responses to anxiety, clients escape from reality into hallucination and/or delusional behavior.

87. **1.** BuSpar must be taken as a maintenance drug, not as a prn response to symptoms. Improvement may be noted in 7–10 days, but it may take 3 to 4 weeks to note therapeutic effects.

88. **2.** The depressant effects of alcohol and alprazolan will be potentiated and may cause harmful sedation.

89. **1.** Confronting fear diminishes the phobic response and the anticipatory anxiety that precedes it.

90. **3.** This is the best action because the nurse is conveying her support. Later, she would need to further assess the client's fear of elevators and respond accordingly.

91. **2.** Parental role conflict is the state in which a parent experiences role confusion and conflict in response to crisis. Loss of economic base constitutes a crisis state.

92. **1.** The nurse should remove the client from the group to provide a safe environment for her and others. The nurse should stay with the client and provide comfort and reality orientation.

93. **3.** There is comorbidity between Tourette's syndrome and obsessive-compulsive disorder.

94. **2.** Improvement in relation to delusional content includes a reduction in the disturbing quality of the delusions and the client's ability to control and/or not respond to them.

95. **4.** Symptoms of post-traumatic stress disorder range from emotional ''numbness'' to vivid nightmares in which the traumatic event is recalled.

96. **1.** Thought stopping techniques, flooding, and response prevention have proven effective in treating clients with OCD. Clients may shout or think ''stop'' or snap a rubber band on their wrist to dismiss the obsessive thought.

97. **2.** If the client adheres to the unit schedule, it is likely that her obsessions and compulsive rituals have lessened. They no longer preoccupy her to the point of interfering with activities.

98. **1.** Post-trauma response is the state of an individual experiencing a sustained painful response to an overwhelming traumatic event.

99. **3.** Cognitive treatment for PTSD includes redefining the event by considering benefits of the experience and finding meaning in the experience.

100. **2.** The client's behavior is indicative of personal identity disturbance related to a traumatic event, the rape. The client is unable to recall her identity, which is a factor in dissociative disorders. The person loses the ability to integrate consciousness, memory, identity, or motor behavior.

101. **2.** This lack of concern is identified as ''la belle indifference'' and is often a clue that the problem may be psychological rather than physical.

102. 4. Hypochondriasis is excessive preoccupation with one's physical health, without organic pathology.

103. 1. This is an appropriate long-term goal related to the client's ineffective coping (use of conversion symptom, paralysis) related to unresolved conflicts and anxiety.

104. 3. This goal is related to the client's impaired social interaction in response to his preoccupation with illness.

105. 1. In dissociative amnesia, an individual is unable to recall important personal information such as name, occupation, and relatives.

106. 3. Self-mutilation is characteristic of borderline personality disorder.

107. 4. A safe environment for the client is a priority.Her self-mutilation, poor impulse control, and temper are characteristic of persons with borderline personality disorder who have self-directed violence.

108. 4. The client's acting out and demanding behavior indicates her need for ego boundaries and control, which the nurse provides.

109. 3. Clients with borderline personality disorder frequently engage in impulsive suicidal or self-mutilating behaviors. The behavior described in choice 3 indicates less "acting-out" of feelings and less impulsiveness in response to more effective coping.

110. 4. This is an appropriate short-term goal in relation to his use of manipulative behavior to meet his needs.

111. 3. This would indicate that the client may be improving related to recognizing his manipulative behavior. This is a first step in reducing the need for manipulation and attaining more effective coping strategies.

3

Psychologic Aspects of Physical Illness

■ STRESS-RELATED DISORDERS

Overview

1. Actual physiologic change in structure/function of organ or system
2. May be referred to as psychosomatic or psychophysiologic disorders
3. Theorized that client's response to stress is a factor in etiology of disease
4. Stress/anxiety not the sole cause but may be a causative factor in the development/exacerbation of physical symptoms
5. See Table 3-1 for types of disorders with a stress component.

Assessment

A. Health history, family history
B. Physical symptoms
C. Social/cultural considerations
D. Coping behaviors

Analysis

Nursing diagnoses for stress-related disorders may include any nursing diagnosis specific to the physiologic problem as well as
A. Ineffective coping
B. Deficient knowledge
C. Health-seeking behaviors

Planning and Implementation

Goals

Client will
A. Receive appropriate treatment for any physical symptoms (e.g., maintenance of blood pressure within normal range).

TABLE 3-1   Types of Stress-Related Disorders

Systems	Examples
Respiratory	Asthma, common cold
Circulatory	Hypertension, migraine headaches
Digestive	Peptic ulcers, colitis
Skin	Hives, dermatitis
Musculoskeletal	Rheumatoid arthritis, chronic backache
Nervous	Fatigue
Endocrine	Dysmenorrhea, diabetes mellitus

B. Recognize relationship of stress to physical symptom(s).
C. Acknowledge coping patterns that may affect recurrence of physical symptoms.
D. Recognize relationship of self-concept, self-esteem, role performance to disorder.
E. Develop alternative coping behaviors.

Interventions
A. Provide nursing care specific to physical symptoms.
B. Establish nurse-client relationship.
C. Encourage discussion of psychosocial problems.
D. Explain relationship of stress to physiologic symptoms.
E. Encourage client to devise alternative coping behaviors, changes in environment, attitude.
F. Role play new behaviors with client.

Evaluation
A. Goals specific to client's physical symptoms have been met.
B. Client
   1. Is able to relate stress to physical symptoms.
   2. Develops alternative coping behaviors.
   3. Engages in role playing of new behaviors.

> **DELEGATION TIP**
>
> F ederal law requires the reporting of all suspected child abuse to Child Protective Services.

■ VICTIMS OF ABUSE

Overview

A. Abuse is physical or sexual assault, emotional abuse, or neglect.
B. Victims are helpless or powerless to prevent the assault on their bodies or personalities.
C. Sometimes victims blame themselves for the assault.
D. The abusers often blame the victims, have poor impulse control, and use their power (physical strength or weapon) to subject victims to their assaults.
E. Victims include children, spouse, elderly, or rape victims; each will be described separately.

Child Abuse

Overview

A. Over one million cases reported each year
B. Suspected child abuse must be reported
C. Abusing adults (parents) often have been victims of abuse, substance abusers, have poor impulse control
D. Battered-child syndrome: multiple traumas inflicted by adult
E. Sexual abuse/incest: common types of child abuse
F. Health care workers often experience negative feelings toward abuser

Assessment

A. Physical signs/behaviors or physical/sexual abuse (see Table 3-2)
B. Signs of neglect: hunger, poor hygiene/nutrition, fatigue
C. Signs of emotional abuse: habitual behaviors (thumb sucking, rocking, head banging), conduct/learning disorders

Analysis

A. Situational low self-esteem
B. Fear
C. Pain
D. Altered parenting
E. Post-trauma response
F. Powerlessness
G. High risk for injury

TABLE 3-2 Symptoms of Child Abuse

Physical Abuse	Sexual Abuse
Pattern of bruises/welts	Pain/itching of genitals
Burns (cigarette, scalds, rope)	Bruised/bleeding genitals
Unexplained fractures/dislocations	Stains/blood on underwear
Withdrawn or aggressive behavior	Withdrawn or aggressive behavior
Unusual fear of parent/desire to please parent	Unusual sexual behaviors

Planning and Implementation

A. Goals
   1. Client (child) will be safe until home assessment made by child welfare agency.
   2. Child will participate with nurse (therapist) for emotional support.
   3. Client (parent(s)) will be able to contact agencies to deal with own rage/helplessness.
   4. Parent(s) will participate in therapy (group or other required).
B. Interventions
   1. Provide nursing care specific to physical/emotional symptoms.
   2. Conduct interview in private with child and parent(s) separated.
   3. Inform parent(s) of requirement to report suspected abuse.
   4. Do not probe for information or try to prove abuse.
   5. Be supportive and nonjudgmental.
   6. Provide referrals for assistance and therapy.
C. Evaluation
   1. Physical symptoms have been treated.
   2. Child safety has been ensured.
   3. Parent(s) have agreed to seek help.

Spouse Abuse

Overview

A. Estimates of five million women assaulted by mate each year
B. Stages
   1. Tension builds: verbal abuse, minor physical assaults

      a. Abuser: often reduces tension with alcohol/drugs
      b. Abused: blames self
  2. Acute battering: brutal beating
      a. Abuser: does not recall incident
      b. Abused: depersonalizes, may seek separation/divorce
      c. Both parties in shock
  3. Honeymoon: make-up stage
      a. Abuser: apologizes and promises to control self
      b. Abused: feels loved/needed; forgives/believes abuser
  4. Cycle repeats with subsequent battering, usually more severe

Assessment

A. Headache
B. Injury to face, head, body, genitals
C. Reports "accidents"
D. Symptoms of severe anxiety
E. Depression
F. Insomnia

Analysis

A. Risk for injury
B. Anxiety
C. Pain
D. Disabled family coping
E. Ineffective coping
F. Spiritual distress

Planning and Implementation

Goals: Client will
A. Admit self and/or children are victims of abuse
B. Describe plan(s) for own/children's safety
C. Name agencies that will assist in maintaining a safe environment
Interventions
A. Crisis stage
  1. Provide safe environment
  2. Treatment of physical injuries; document
  3. Encourage verbalization of actual home environment
  4. Provide referral to shelters
  5. Encourage decision making
B. Rebuilding stage: therapy (individual, family and/or group)

Evaluation

Client will be protected from further injury.

Elder Abuse

Overview

A. Estimates one-half million to over one million cases per year.
B. Women, over age 70, with some physical/ psychological disability are most frequent victims.
C. Neglect is most common, followed by physical abuse, financial exploitation, and sexual abuse/abandonment.
D. Victims do not always report abuse because of fear of more abuse/ abandonment by caretaker(s).

Assessment

A. Malnutrition
B. Poor hygiene, decubiti
C. Omission of medication/overmedication
D. Welts, bruises, fractures

Analysis

A. Risk for injury
B. Fear
C. Anxiety
D. Imbalanced nutrition: less than body requirements
E. Powerlessness
F. Situational low self-esteem

Planning and Implementation

Goals
A. Client will be free from injury.
B. Client will receive adequate nutrition, hydration, prescribed medication.
C. Client will notify nurse if further abuse takes place.
D. Caregiver will verbalize plans to meet own needs.
E. Caregiver will seek assistance to meet client's needs when necessary.
Interventions
A. Refer to state laws for reporting elder abuse and nurse's liability.
B. Obtain client's consent for treatment and/or transfer.
C. Document physical/emotional condition of client.
D. Refer client/caregiver to agencies for assistance.
E. Encourage client and caregiver to discuss problems.
F. Encourage communication between client and caregiver.

Evaluation

A. Client will remain free of injury, effects of neglect.
B. Caregiver will utilize support systems for self.

Rape

Overview

A. Estimates of occurrence vary; only 10% reported
B. Most victims are female between ages of 15 and 24 years
C. Response to rape
   1. Shock: panic to overly controlled
   2. Outward adjustment: "manages" life but may make drastic changes (e.g., moves, leaves school/job)
   3. Integration: acknowledges response (e.g., depression, fear, rage)

Assessment

A. Physical injury
B. Emotional response: controlled/hysterical

Analysis

A. Rape trauma syndrome
   1. Compound reaction: immediate to 2 weeks (anger, fear, self-blame)
   2. Long-term: nightmares, phobias, seeks support
B. Silent reaction: anxiety, changes in relationships with men, physical distress, phobias
C. Post-trauma response

Planning and Implementation

Goals: Client will
A. Express response to assault
B. Verbalize plan to handle immediate needs
C. Seek assistance from rape counselor
D. Discuss need for follow-up counseling
E. Report (long-term) reduction of physical and emotional symptoms.
Interventions
A. Give emotional support in nonjudgmental manner.
B. Maintain confidentiality: client must give consent for reporting rape and for medical examination.
C. Listen to client, encourage expression of feelings.
D. Document physical findings. Put evidentiary garments in paper bag.
E. Provide referral to rape counselor and follow-up care.

Evaluation

A. Client seeks support from family/agencies.
B. Client verbalizes emotional response to rape.
C. Long-term: client reports return to prerape lifestyle.

■ CRITICAL ILLNESS

Overview

A. Individuals in critical life-threatening situations have realistic fears of death or of permanent loss of function.
B. Clients and their families may respond to these crises with denial, anger, hostility, withdrawal, guilt, and/or panic.
C. Loss of control and a sense of powerlessness can be overwhelming and detrimental to chance of recovery.

Assessment

A. Physiologic needs (first priority)
B. Anxiety level of client/family
C. Client/family fears
D. Coping behaviors of client/family
E. Social and cultural considerations

Analysis

Nursing diagnoses for the psychologic component of critical illness may include
A. Anxiety
B. Hopelessness
C. Ineffective coping
D. Deficient knowledge
E. Fear
F. Powerlessness

Planning and Implementation

Goals

A. Client will
 1. Receive treatment for physiologic problems.
 2. Experience decrease in level of anxiety/fear.
 3. Discuss anxiety/fears with nurse.
B. Family will
 1. Be informed of client's condition on regular basis.
 2. Discuss anxiety/fears with nurse.
 3. Provide appropriate support to client.

Interventions

A. Provide nursing care specific to physiologic problems.
B. Stay with client.
C. Explain all procedures slowly, clearly, concisely.
D. Provide opportunities for client to discuss fears.

E. Provide opportunities for client to make decisions, have as much control as possible.
F. Encourage family to ask questions.
G. Recognize negative family responses as coping behaviors.
H. Encourage family members to support each other and client.

Evaluation

A. Goals specific to client's physiologic status have been met.
B. Client
  1. Demonstrates a decrease in anxious behaviors.
  2. Is able to express fears verbally.
  3. Has participated in decisions whenever possible.
C. Family members
  1. Have discussed fears.
  2. Demonstrate support for each other and for client.

■ CHRONIC ILLNESS

Overview

A. Chronic illnesses, such as diabetes mellitus, multiple sclerosis, or illnesses/injuries resulting in loss of function or loss of a body part necessitate adaptation to the inherent changes imposed.
B. Clients/families may respond to the losses associated with chronic illness with a variety of behaviors and defenses, including recurrent depression, anger and hostility, denial, or acceptance.

Assessment and Analysis

Same as stress-related disorders as well as
A. Ineffective coping
B. Risk for violence, self-directed
C. Spiritual distress

Planning and Intervention

Goals

A. Client will
  1. Receive appropriate treatment for any physiologic symptoms.
  2. Be able/willing to discuss responses to illness.
  3. Recognize effect of illness on aspects of self-concept.
  4. Develop realistic plans for activities and role functions.
  5. Contract with nurse to report depression/ suicidal ideation.
B. Family will
  1. Be able to discuss responses to client illness.
  2. Develop plans to deal with alterations in client's behaviors and functions.

NURSING ALERT
Depression, anxiety, and psychosis may occur as the disease progresses.

Interventions

A. Provide nursing care specific to physiologic problems.
B. Develop nurse/client relationship through active listening, acceptance of positive and negative client responses.
C. Encourage client to plan activities within present capabilities.
D. Provide information about illness, suggestions for activities.
E. Contract with client to request support in times of depression and to report suicidal ideation.
F. Encourage family members to discuss their response to client's illness.
G. Be accepting and nonjudgmental of negative responses (e.g., anger, hopelessness).
H. Support family efforts to develop plans for their participation in client's care.

Evaluation

A. Client
  1. Receives appropriate treatment for any physiologic problems.
  2. Recognizes/discusses positive and negative responses to illness.
  3. Understands effects of feelings about body image, self-esteem, role function.
  4. Agrees to report depression or suicidal thoughts.
B. Family
  1. Discusses positive and negative responses to client's illness.
  2. Plans/engages in appropriate activities with client.

■ AIDS

Overview

A. In the United States, many thousands of reported cases and deaths, estimates between 1 and 2 million infected.
B. Highest risk populations: homosexual/bisexual men, IV drug users and their sexual partners, hemophiliacs, newborns from infected mothers, and black females between the ages of 15 and 44 years.
C. Approximately 60% of persons with AIDS develop neurological symptoms.
D. Health care workers may have difficulty caring for these clients because of fear of contagion, knowledge deficit, bias against lifestyle, or burnout.
E. Families/partners will require support, education, and/or counseling.

NURSING ALERT

All health care workers must implement standard precautions.

Assessment

A. Physical symptoms
 1. Fever
 2. Fatigue
 3. Weight loss
 4. Diarrhea
 5. Opportunistic infections
B. Neurological and emotional responses
 1. Depression
 2. Panic disorders
 3. Paranoid reaction
 4. HIV dementia complex
C. See AIDS for other physical assessment findings.

Analysis

A. Anxiety
B. Fear
C. Ineffective denial
D. Anticipatory grieving
E. Ineffective coping
F. Powerlessness
G. Risk for violence, self-directed
H. Social isolation

Planning and Implementation

Goals

A. Client will
 1. Communicate responses (physical and psychologic) to disease process
 2. Maintain ADL as long as possible
 3. Report suicidal ideation/impulses
B. Family/partners will
 1. Seek support and education relating to care of HIV-positive client
 2. Communicate responses to client's illness to nurse/support group
C. Health care workers will
 1. Discuss feelings of homophobia, addictophobia, and fear of infection
 2. Attend groups for education and support

CLIENT TEACHING CHECKLIST

Educate the client and family regarding

- Coping skills
- Stress management
- Participation in treatment planning
- Support group
- Nutrition
- Self-care

Interventions

A. Monitor cognitive and affective domain.
B. Encourage communication of fears and concerns.
C. Maintain nonjudgmental attitude.
D. Assist client/family through grieving process.
E. Provide opportunities for decision making to client and/or caregivers.

Evaluation

A. Client participates in care decisions.
B. Client and caregivers discuss responses to illness.
C. Client expresses anger but does not harm self.

■ DEATH AND DYING

Overview

A. One of the most difficult issues in nursing practice
B. Often difficult for nurses to maintain objectivity because of identification and response to death based on own value system and personal experiences

Assessment

A. Stage of dying (Kubler-Ross); see Table 3-3
B. Physical discomfort
C. Emotional reaction (withdrawal, anger, acceptance) and stage of dying
D. Desire to discuss impending death, value of own life
E. Level of consciousness
F. Family needs

	TABLE 3-3
	Stages of Dying

1.	Denial and isolation
2.	Anger
3.	Bargaining
4.	Depression
5.	Acceptance

Analysis

Nursing diagnoses for the dying client may include

A. Anxiety
B. Pain
C. Ineffective coping
D. Fear
E. Anticipatory grieving
F. Hopelessness
G. Impaired mobility
H. Powerlessness
I. Self-care deficit
J. Social isolation

Planning and Implementation

Goals

A. Client will
   1. Be maintained in optimum comfort.
   2. Not be alone.
   3. Have opportunity to discuss what death means and to progress through stages of dying.
B. Family will have opportunity to be with client as much as they desire.

Interventions

A. Recognize clients/families have own way of dealing with death and dying.
B. Support clients/families as they work through dying process.
C. Accept negative responses from clients/families.
D. Encourage clients/families to discuss feelings related to death and dying.
E. Support staff and seek support for self when dealing with dying client and grieving family.

Evaluation

A. Client
   1. Takes opportunity to discuss feelings about impending death and eventually acknowledges inevitable outcome.

    2. Is comfortable and participates in self-care for as long as possible.
B. Family discusses feelings about loss of loved one.

■ GRIEF AND MOURNING
Overview
A. Response to loss (person, body part, role)
B. Biologic, psychologic, social implications
C. Family system effects
D. Mourning is process to resolve grief
    1. Shock, disbelief are short term
    2. Resentment, anger
    3. Concentration on loss
        a. Possible auditory, visual hallucinations
        b. Possible guilt
        c. Possible fear of becoming mentally ill
    4. Despair, depression
    5. Detachment from loss
    6. Renewed interest, investment in others/interests

Assessment
A. Weight loss
B. Sleep disturbance
C. Thoughts centered on loss
D. Dependency, withdrawal, anger, guilt
E. Suicide potential

Analysis
A. Ineffective coping
B. Hopelessness
C. Sleep pattern disturbance
D. Disturbed thought processes
E. Risk for violence, self-directed

Planning and Implementation
Goals
Client/family will
A. Discuss responses to loss.
B. Resume normal sleeping/eating patterns.
C. Resume ADL as they accept loss.

Interventions
A. Encourage client/family to express feelings.
B. Accept negative feelings/defenses.

C. Employ empathic listening.
D. Explain mourning process and relate to client/family responses.
E. Refer client/family to support groups.

Evaluation

Client/family
A. Express feelings.
B. Progress through mourning process.
C. Seek necessary support groups.

REVIEW QUESTIONS

1. An 18-month-old has been admitted for second-degree burns surrounding the genital area. Her mother told the nurse that the child grabbed for the hot coffee cup and spilled it on herself. The nurse is required by law to

    1. testify in court on the injuries.

    2. report suspected child abuse.

    3. have the mother arrested.

    4. refer the mother to counseling.

2. A toddler was admitted for second-degree burns surrounding the genital area. Her mother told the nurse that the child grabbed the hot coffee cup and spilled it on herself. The toddler's mother is 17 years old. In which of the areas would the nurse provide health teaching?

    1. Normal growth and development.

    2. Bonding techniques.

    3. How to childproof the apartment.

    4. Parenting skills.

3. A young woman was returning home from work late and was sexually assaulted. She was brought to the emergency room upset and crying. The nurse's main goal in caring for her is to

    1. assist her in crisis.

    2. notify the police of the alleged assault.

    3. understand she will have a long recovery period.

    4. provide support and comfort.

4. The nurse is caring for a young woman who was sexually assaulted. Which of the following is indicative of successful adjustment to the trauma?

    1. She moves to another city.

    2. She resumes her work and activities.

3. She takes classes in the martial arts.

4. She remains silent about the assault.

5. A young man has recently begun experiencing forgetfulness, disorientation, and occasional lapses in memory. The client was diagnosed with AIDS dementia. His family began sobbing on hearing the diagnosis. The nurse's initial response would be

1. "You must never give up hope."

2. "He was in a high-risk group for AIDS."

3. "I can understand your grief."

4. "This must be very difficult for you."

6. The nurse is planning care for a young man who has AIDS dementia. The primary goal in his care is to

1. enhance the quality of life.

2. teach him about AIDS.

3. discuss his future goals.

4. provide him with comfort and support.

7. One of the major fears experienced by people with AIDS is

1. dying.

2. debilitation.

3. stigma.

4. poverty.

8. A school nurse is assessing a second grade child for symptoms of sexual abuse. Which of the following behavioral symptoms would support the possibility of sexual abuse?

1. Enuresis, impulsivity, decline in school performance.

2. Thumb sucking, isolating self from peers on playground, excessive fearfulness.

3. Hyperactivity, rocking, isolating self from peers on playground.

4. Stuttering, rocking, impulsivity.

9. A 21-year-old college student is seen in the ER following an incident of date rape. During the nursing assessment, the client describes the entire chain of events with a blank facial expression. She ends her comments by saying, "It's like it didn't happen to me at all." Which of the following statements most accurately explains that patient's reaction?

1. This client is using dissociation/isolation as a defense mechanism to cope with the attack.

2. This client is using denial as a defense mechanism to cope with the attack.

3. This client is in the shock phase of a crisis and is repressing feelings associated with the traumatic event.

4. This client is using reaction formation to manage the hostility she feels toward the attacker.

10. A 38-year-old mother of three children is seen in the medical clinic with complaints of chronic fatigue. The woman looks sad, makes only brief eye contact, and startles easily. The nurse acknowledges these observations and the woman says, "My husband has started to hold a gun to my head when I don't do exactly what he wants." Which of the following is the most appropriate response by the nurse?

1. "What is it you won't do that makes him do this?"

2. "Tell me what has influenced your decision to stay with your husband?"

3. "That is abusive behavior; there are resources which can help you."

4. "How often does this happen?"

11. Which of the following statements made by a victim of spouse abuse would indicate to the nurse that the woman was admitting that she was a victim of spouse abuse?

1. "It would be nice to be out of the situation, but I cannot afford to leave. I have no skills."

2. "My husband has never visited me when I've been in the hospital. He even said he will take me out more often."

3. "Last time it happened I tried to talk to his mother. She said he was never like this growing up."

4. "I have the shelter number and I've decided to work on my high school diploma while the kids are in school each day."

12. A 78-year-old male with a history of cancer of the prostate is admitted to the medical unit for the fourth time in 6 weeks. On admission, the client is confused and has a decubitis ulcer the size of a fifty cent piece on the sacral area. The client did not have this breakdown on discharge 10 days ago. The nurse also notes what appear to be friction burns on both wrists. Which of the following nursing diagnosis statements takes priority in the care of this patient?

1. Impaired Skin integrity.

2. Disturbed thought processes.

3. Ineffective health maintenance.

4. Risk for injury.

13. A 27-year-old is admitted to the medical unit with severe abdominal pain, dehydration, and renal insufficiency associated with substance abuse. The patient's admitting chest X-ray shows diffuse interstitial infiltrates and the physician asks that the client give consent for HIV testing. The client consents and the test returns positive. After learning of the positive results, the client says to the nurse, "I never thought this would happen to me. I don't know if I can go through this." Which of the following nursing diagnosis statements is of highest priority for this patient?

   1. Anticipatory grieving.

   2. Risk for infection.

   3. Risk for self-directed violence.

   4. Thought process, altered.

14. The nurse is changing the dressing on a client who has had a modified radical mastectomy 2 days ago. The client refuses to look in the direction of the nurse or the operative site. The nurse notices a tear running down the client's cheek. Which of the following responses would most appropriately facilitate the client's grief resolution?

   1. "You look very sad, it might help you feel better if you let yourself cry."

   2. "Tell me what's the worst part about losing your breast."

   3. "Everything is going to be all right; you can be fitted for a new bra and no one will notice."

   4. "Are you crying because you are concerned about how your partner will respond?"

15. A 42-year-old male is admitted to the medical unit for insertion of an access site for hemodialysis. The client relates that his transplant graft failed, he has lost his job due to corporate downsizing, and his wife left him recently. He has now moved back into his parents' home. Which of the following nursing diagnosis statements takes priority in planning nursing care for this client?

   1. Fluid volume deficit.

   2. Ineffective denial.

   3. Ineffective tissue perfusion; renal.

   4. Powerlessness.

16. The condition of a client diagnosed with chronic obstructive pulmonary disease (COPD) and cor pulmonale is deteriorating. The client is very hypoxemic, obtunded, and easily fatigued by any activity. The nurse who has been working with this client throughout this hospitalization is repositioning the client. Which of the following remarks made by the client indicates that the client has come to terms with death?

1. "It is finally spring and that is my favorite time of year."
2. "Am I going to die?"
3. "I'm very tired, but content and ready to go."
4. "I'm feeling stronger by the moment today."

17. A family member whose mother is terminally ill asks to speak to the nurse. Which of the following statements made by this family member should indicate to the nurse that this family member understands the emotional response to death and dying?

1. "Mother seems very comfortable; so we're able to recall some of our good times spent together."
2. "My mother is irate because she says you all told her she had to have an advanced directive."
3. "My mother is talking about redoing her bedroom when she's discharged. Doesn't she know she's dying?"
4. "My mother is crying so much these days. Where's all this sadness coming from?"

ANSWERS AND RATIONALES

1. 2. Legal statutes require health professionals to report suspected cases of child abuse. The burn pattern described is consistent with being placed in a tub of very hot water.

2. 4. Because the toddler's mother is only 17 years old, she needs information and role modeling on how to provide an emotionally and physically safe environment for her child. This response is more inclusive and includes the other responses.

3. 1. A sexual assault is a crisis situation that requires crisis intervention.

4. 2. The goal of adjustment is to have the woman return to her precrisis level of functioning.

5. 4. AIDS is an illness that generates intense emotional reactions and fears. Acknowledging these feelings allows the family to discuss them with the nurse in a nonthreatening environment.

6. 1. Because the client's illness has no cure and the progression is dependent on the body system affected, the primary goal is to ensure his personal dignity and make plans to fulfill personal goals.

7. 2. Research has found that many clients with AIDS are most fearful of the debilitating effects of the disease.

8. 2. Behavioral symptoms of children who are victims of sexual abuse include: regression (thumb sucking would be regressive behavior in a

second grade child who is probably around 7 years old), disturbed sleep patterns, clinging behaviors, lack of peer friendships, sexual acting out, running away or threats to do so, and suicide attempts.

9. 1. One of the defense mechanisms that a person can use to manage the anxiety associated with an attack/rape is dissociation/isolation in which the client strips an event of its emotional significance and affective content.141. 3.This response identifies the husband's behavior as abusive and offers help for the wife if she is ready to consider other options. It does not cast judgment on her or question why she stays.

10. 3. This response identifies the husband's behavior as abusive and offers help for the wife if she is ready to consider other options. It does not cast judgment on her or question why she stays.

11. 4. This statement acknowledges that the victim has admitted the need for protection in case of emergency and is making plans to work on establishing some degree of autonomy, which is a factor that keeps many women in abusive relationships.

12. 4. The highest priority for this client based on the available data is the increased risk for injury because of confusion. The nurse's immediate concern must be the client's safety in the present environment.

13. 3. Based on the patient's comment, the highest priority of care for this client immediately is the risk of suicide. He states he doesn't know if he can go through this. Suicide is a common reaction of persons who learn they are HIV-positive, which is associated with stigma and many losses. The client does not have a history of positive coping, which increases the risk of suicide.

14. 1. This acknowledges the client's mood and gives her permission to cry. Crying puts the client in touch with the sadness/pain over the loss. Offering permission to cry facilitates expression of feelings related to the loss.

15. 4. Powerlessness, or feelings of uncertainty about the future, may be present in this client due to the uncertainty about his future in several areas: job, another transplant, long-term hemodialysis, reconciliation in his marriage, whether he will have to be dependent on parents long term, and concern about their own possible declining health.

16. 3. This response indicates that the client is exhausted and ready to let the natural processes take their course. The client is at peace.

17. 1. This statement indicates that the family member and mother have been able to reminisce about good times together, acknowledging that there may be few remaining times to share these memories. This sharing indicates both have accepted death of mother and its finality.

Appendices Table of Contents

Appendix A: Theorists Stages of Development

Stage	Age	Characteristics
Freud's Stages of Development		
Oral stage	0-12 months	Oral gratification, sucking
Anal stage	1-3 years	Rectal gratification, control of bowel movements
Phallic/oedipal stage	3-6 years	Genital fixation and concentration
Latency stage	6-11 years	Repression of sexual feelings and memories
Puberty	11 years on	Rise in sexual energy, independence from parents
Erikson's Stages of Development		
Trust versus mistrust	0-18 months	Development of trust
Autonomy versus shame and doubt	18 months-3 years	Exercise of choice and self-determination

Continued

Stage	Age	Characteristics
Initiative versus guilt	3-6 years	Exploration and daring
Industry versus inferiority	6-11 years	Mastery of social and cognitive skills
Identity versus role confusion	11-20 years	Development of identity
Intimacy versus isolation	18-25 years	Mutuality and intimacy with another person
Generativity versus stagnation	21-45 years	Productivity through caring for and guiding children
Ego integrity versus despair	45 years to death	Internal struggle and life review

Piaget's Stage Theory of Cognitive Development

Sensorimotor intelligence	0-2 years	
Preoperational thought	2-7 years	
Concrete operations	7-11 years	
Formal operations	11 years to adulthood	

Appendix B: Milieu Elements and Interventions across the Life Span

	CHILD	ADOLESCENT	ADULT	GERIATRIC
1.Containment (Safety) (Continuum of mental health services)	• Close supervision • Time out • Seclusion Mental and physical status exams Health education/parenting classes as needed Discharge planning Identify cultural needs and integrate into treatment planning	• Flexible supervision • Quiet time • Seclusion • Suicide alert Mental and physical status exams Discharge planning Identify cultural needs and integrate into treatment planning	• Flexible supervision • Quiet time • Medication Mental and physical status exams Discharge planning Identify cultural needs and integrate into treatment planning	• Close supervision • Suicide alert • Provide medical care Emotional support Mental and physical status exams Discharge planning Identify cultural needs and integrate into treatment planning

Continued

129

	CHILD	ADOLESCENT	ADULT	GERIATRIC
2. Support (Continuum of mental health services)	• Give attention • Reassure • Direct • Redirect • Praise • Touch* • Hug* Use ACT, intensive case management Facilitate psychosocial rehabilitation	• Give attention • Reassure • Encourage • Educate • Praise Use ACT, intensive case management Facilitate psychosocial rehabilitation	• Reassurance • Encouragement • Educate • Praise • Give feedback Use ACT, intensive case management Facilitate psychosocial rehabilitation	• Give attention • Reassure • Encourage • Give direction • Provide comfort measures Use ACT, intensive case management Facilitate psychosocial rehabilitation
3. Structure (Continuum of mental health services)	• Schedule activity: short time periods Enhance activities of daily living skills	• Schedule activity: + free time DBT model for personality disorders	• Schedule activity: + free time DBT model for personality disorders	• Schedule activity: with rest periods DBT model for personality disorders

4. Involvement (Continuum of mental health services)	• Allow choices • Teach problem solving Focus on symptom management and medication adherence Foster recreational activities and social skills training in community	• Expect active participation • Teach decision making Focus on symptom management and medication adherence Foster recreational activities and social skills training in community	• Expect the client to participate in treatment planning Focus on symptom management and medication adherence Foster recreational activities and social skills training in community	• Encourage social activity Focus on symptom management and medication adherence Foster recreational activities and social skills training in community
5. Open Communication (Continuum of mental health services)	• Teach to name feelings • Encourage verbal expression of feelings • Develop trust Consultation with various services Timely and accurate documentation	• Avoid secret keeping • Discourage manipulation • Encourage verbal sharing with peers	• Explain that confidentiality is unit based • Encourage appropriate self-disclosure	• Encourage to share memories • Encourage to acknowledge loss and adaptation

Continued

	CHILD	ADOLESCENT	ADULT	GERIATRIC
6. Family and Community (Continuum of mental health services)	• Avoid abrupt separations • Provide emotional support ACT and intensive case management models Integrate cultural considerations	• Strong school-unit collaboration ACT and intensive case management models Integrate cultural considerations	• Assist with return to work ACT and intensive case management models Integrate cultural considerations	• Assist with placement/home care decisions ACT and intensive case management models Integrate cultural considerations
7. Physical Environment (Continuum of mental health services)	• Age-sized furniture • Client rooms easily observed • Pleasant sensory stimulation	• Group activity areas • Quiet areas • Music areas	• Group activity areas • Quiet areas • Attractive furniture	• Safe mobility aids • Many orientation cues

*Only with client consent

Note: Data from "Effective Treatment for Mental Disorders in Children and Adolescents," by B. J. Burns, K. Hoagwood, and P. J. Mrazek, 1999, *Clinical Child and Family Psychology, 2*, pp. 199–254; "Establishing a Therapeutic Milieu with Adolescents," by D. Creedy and M. Crowe, 1996, *Australian and New Zealand Journal of Mental Health Nursing, 5*, pp. 84–89; "Effects of Social Skills Training and Social Milieu Treatment of Schizophrenia," by D. J. Dobson, G. McDougall, J. Busheikin, and J. Aldous, 1995, *Psychiatric Services, 46*, pp. 376–380; "Milieu Management for Traumatized Youngers," by L. Lawson, 1998, *Child and Adolescent Psychiatric Nursing, 11*, pp. 99–106; and "Milieu Therapy for Short Stay Units: A Transformed Practice Theory," by E. A. LeCuyer, 1992, *Archives of Psychiatric Nursing, 6(2)*, pp. 108–116.

Appendix C: Nanda Nursing Diagnoses 2005–2006

Activity Intolerance

Risk for Activity Intolerence

Impaired Adjustment

Ineffective Airway Clearance

Latex Allergy Response

Risk for Latex Allergy Response

Anxiety

Death Anxiety

Risk for Aspiration

Risk for Impaired Parent/Infant/Child Attachment

Autonomic Dysreflexia

Risk for Autonomic Dysreflexia

Disturbed Body Image

Risk for Imbalanced Body Temperature

Bowel Incontinence

Effective Breastfeeding

Ineffective Breastfeeding

Interrupted Breastfeeding

Ineffective Breathing Pattern

Decreased Cardiac Output

Caregiver Role Strain

Risk for Caregiver Role Strain

Impaired Verbal Communication

Readiness for Enhanced Communication

Decisional Conflict (Specify)

Parental Role Conflict

Acute Confusion

Chronic Confusion

Constipation

Perceived Constipation

Risk for Constipation

Defensive Coping

Ineffective Coping

Readiness for Enhanced Coping

Ineffective Community Coping

Readiness for Enhanced Community Coping

Compromised Family Coping

Disabled Family Coping

Readiness for Enhanced Family Coping

Risk for Sudden Infant Death Syndrome

Ineffective Denial

Impaired Dentition

Risk for Delayed Development

Diarrhea

Risk for Disuse Syndrome

Deficient Diversional Activity

Energy Field Disturbance

Impaired Environmental
  Interpretation Syndrome

Adult Failure to Thrive

Risk for Falls

Dysfunctional Family Processes:
  Alcoholism

Interrupted Family Processes

Readiness for Enhanced Family
  Processes

Fatigue

Fear

Readiness for Enhanced Fluid Balance

Deficient Fluid Volume

Excess Fluid Volume

Risk for Deficient Fluid Volume

Risk for Imbalanced Fluid Volume

Impaired Gas Exchange

Anticipatory Grieving

Dysfunctional Grieving

Risk for Dysfunctional Grieving

Delayed Growth and Development

Risk for Disproportionate Growth

Ineffective Health Maintenance

Health-Seeking Behaviors (Specify)

Impaired Home Maintenance

Hopelessness

Hyperthermia

Hypothermia

Disturbed Personal Identity

Functional Urinary Incontinence

Reflex Urinary Incontinence

Stress Urinary Incontinence

Total Urinary Incontinence

Urge Urinary Incontinence

Risk for Urge Urinary Incontinence

Disorganized Infant Behavior

Risk for Disorganized Infant Behavior

Readiness for Enhanced Organized
  Infant Behavior

Ineffective Infant Feeding Pattern

Risk for Infection

Risk for Injury

Risk for Perioperative-Positioning
  Injury

Decreased Intracranial Adaptive
  Capacity

Deficient Knowledge

Readiness for Enhanced Knowledge
  (Specify)

Risk for Loneliness

Impaired Memory

Impaired Bed Mobility

Impaired Physical Mobility

Impaired Wheelchair Mobility

Nausea

Unilateral Neglect

Noncompliance

Imbalanced Nutrition: Less than Body
  Requirements

Readiness for Enhanced Nutrition

Risk for Imbalanced Nutrition: More
  than Body Requirements

Impaired Oral Mucous Membrane

Acute Pain

Chronic Pain

Readiness for Enhanced Parenting

Impaired Parenting

Risk for Impaired Parenting

Risk for Peripheral Neurovascular
  Dysfunction

Risk for Poisoning

Post-Trauma Syndrome

Powerlessness

Risk for Powerlessness

Ineffective Protection

Rape-Trauma Syndrome

Rape-Trauma Syndrome: Compound
  Reaction

Rape-Trauma Syndrome: Silent
  Reaction

Impaired Religiosity

Readiness for Enhanced Religiosity

Risk for Impaired Religiosity

Relocation Stress Syndrome

Risk for Relocation Stress Syndrome

Ineffective Role Performance

Sedentary Life Style

Bathing/Hygiene Self-Care Deficit

Dressing/Grooming Self-Care Deficit

Feeding Self-Care Deficit

Toileting Self-Care Deficit

Readiness for Enhanced Self-Concept

Chronic Low Self-Esteem

Situational Low Self-Esteem

Risk for Situational Low Self-Esteem

Self-Mutilation

Risk for Self-Mutilation

Disturbed Sensory Perception
  (Specify: Visual, Auditory,
  Kinesthetic, Gustatory, Tactile,
  Olfactory)

Sexual Dysfunction

Ineffective Sexuality Patterns

Impaired Skin Integrity

Risk for Impaired Skin Integrity

Sleep Deprivation

Disturbed Sleep Pattern

Readiness for Enhanced Sleep

Impaired Social Interaction

Social Isolation

Chronic Sorrow

Spiritual Distress

Risk for Spiritual Distress

Readiness for Enhanced Spiritual
  Well-Being

Risk for Suffocation

Risk for Suicide

Delayed Surgical Recovery

Impaired Swallowing

Effective Therapeutic Regimen
  Management

Ineffective Therapeutic Regimen
  Management

Readiness for Enhanced
  Management of Therapeutic
  Regimen

Ineffective Community Therapeutic
  Regimen Management

Ineffective Family Therapeutic
  Regimen Management

Ineffective Thermoregulation

Disturbed Thought Processes

Impaired Tissue Integrity

Ineffective Tissue Perfusion (Specify
  Type: Renal, Cerebral,
  Cardiopulmonary,
  Gastrointestinal, Peripheral)

Impaired Transfer Ability

Risk for Trauma

Impaired Urinary Elimination

Readiness for Enhanced Urinary
  Elimination

Urinary Retention

Impaired Spontaneous Ventilation

Dysfunctional Ventilatory Weaning
    Response

Risk for Other-Directed Violence

Risk for Self-Directed Violence

Impaired Walking

Wandering

From NANDA International: *Nursing Diagnoses: Definitions & Classification, 2005–2006*, 2005, Philadelphia: Author. Reprinted with permission.

Appendix D: Clinical and Pharmacokinetic Parameters of Antidepressant Medications

GENERIC NAME	BRAND NAME	DOSAGE RANGE (MG/DAY)	HALF-LIFE (HOURS)	ONSET OF CLINICAL EFFECTS	ELIMINATION PERIOD AFTER LAST DOSE	AMINE BLOCKING ACTIVITY*
Tertiary Amines						
Amitriptyline	Elavil	75–200	31–46 (18–44 for nortriptyline)	2–4 weeks for all tertiary amines	≥2 weeks for all tertiary amines	NE (2), 5-HT (4)
Clomipramine	Anafranil	75–300	19–37			NE (2), 5-HT (5)
Doxepin	Sinequan, Adapin	75–300	8–24 (desmethyline)			NE (1), 5-HT (2)

Continued

137

GENERIC NAME	BRAND NAME	DOSAGE RANGE (MG/DAY)	HALF-LIFE (HOURS)	ONSET OF CLINICAL EFFECTS	ELIMINATION PERIOD AFTER LAST DOSE	AMINE BLOCKING ACTIVITY
Imipramine	Tofranil	75–200	11–25 (12–24 for desipramine)			NE (2), 5-HT (4)
Trimipramine	Surmontil	75–200	7–30			NE (1), 5-HT (1)
Secondary Amines						
Amoxapine	Asendin	150–300	8–30 (30 for 7-hydrox and 8-hydrox)	2–4 weeks for all secondary amines	2–4 weeks for all secondary amines	NE (3), 5-HT (2), DA (2)
Desipramine	Norpramin	75–200	12–24			NE (4), 5-HT (2)
Nortriptyline	Aventyl	75–150	18–44			NE (2), 5-HT (3)
Protriptyline	Vivactyl	20–40	67–89			NE (4), 5-HT (2)
Tetracyclic						
Maprotiline	Ludiomil	75–300	21–25	3–7 days 2–3 weeks	2 weeks	NE (3), 5-HT (1)

Triazolopyridine						
Trazodone	Desyrel	50–600	4–9	1–4 weeks	2 weeks	5-HT (3)
Nefazodone	Serzone	300–600	3.5–5			5-HT$_2$ (3), NE (1)
Bicyclics						
Fluoxetine	Prozac	20–80	2–5 days (7–9 days for norfluoxetine)	1–4 days	4 weeks	NE (1), 5-HT (5)
Paroxetine	Paxil	20–50	5–21	Up to 8 weeks	2 weeks	NE (1), DA (1), 5-HT (5)
Sertraline	Zoloft	50–200	24 N-desmethylsertraline (62–104 hours)	Up to 8 weeks	2 weeks	NE (1), DA (1), 5-HT (5)
Aminoketone						
Bupropion	Welbutrin	200–300	8 days (4 weeks for active metabolites)	1–4 weeks	2 weeks	NE (1), 5-HT (1), DA (1)

*NE, norepinepherine; DA, dopamine; 5-T, serotonin. 0 = none, 1 = very weak, 2 = weak, 3 = moderate, 4 = strong, 5 = strongest.

Appendix E: Symptoms Associated with Adverse Effects of Tricyclics and Related Antidepressants

SYSTEM	COMMON SIDE EFFECTS	LESS COMMON SIDE EFFECTS
Cardiovascular	Orthostatic hypotension, tachycardia	Palpitations
Central Nervous	Drowsiness, weakness, fatigue, dizziness, tremors Maprotiline: headaches, restlessness Fluoxetine: headaches, insomnia, anxiety, sexual disturbances Bupropion: agitation, headache, confusion, involuntary movements, ataxia, insomnia, seizures	Confusion, disturbed concentration, decreased memory, electrocardiographic changes
Neurological		Numbness, tingling, paresthesias of extremities, akathisia, ataxia, tremors, extrapyramidal side effects, neuropathy, seizures

Autonomic	Dry mouth, blurred vision, constipation, urinary retention	
	Fluoxetine: excessive sweating	
Gastrointestinal	Maprotiline: nausea	Vomiting, nausea, diarrhea, flatulence
	Trazodone: vomiting	
	Fluoxetine/sertraline: nausea, diarrhea, weight loss, dry mouth	
	Bupropion: nausea, vomiting, abdominal cramps, constipation, dry mouth	
Allergic		Skin rash, pruritus, urticaria, photosensitivity, edema
Respiratory		Pharyngitis, rhinitis, sinusitis

- Psychiatric disorders: Tricyclic and heterocyclic antidepressants can induce a manic episode in clients with bipolar I disorder with and without a prior diagnosed manic episode. These drugs may also exacerbate psychotic disorders. Therefore, it is practical to begin with a low dose in these clients and monitor them for signs of mania or psychosis, or consider another antidepressant.
- Cardiac effects: Caution must be used when administering heterocyclics to clients with cardiovascular disease. In high doses, TCAs may produce arrythmias, sinus tachycardia, flattened T waves, and depressed ST segments and QT intervals. Because the result of these arrythmias prolongs conduction time, preexisting conduction defects contraindicate the use of these antidepressants.
- Risk of overdose: Drug overdoses with these agents can be lethal, especially when combined with alcohol. Because the risk of suicide is also a consideration with depressed clients, until stabilized, they should not be given more than 1 week's supply at a time. In addition, because of the prolonged half-lives of these agents, particularly with overdosing, the risk of cardiac arrythmias is high, requiring cardiac monitoring in the intensive care unit for 3 to 4 days after the overdose attempt (Kaplan & Sadock, 1996).
- Metabolites: One of the breakdown products of the antidepressant amoxapine (Asendin) is loxapine (Loxitane). Because loxapine is an antipsychotic, it carries the risk of extrapyramidal side effects (EPS) and tardive dyskinesia (TD). Many prescribers are reluctant to prescribe this medication for this reason.

Appendix F: Preparation for NCLEX

The future belongs to those who believe in the beauty of their dreams.
(Eleanor Roosevelt)

A new graduate from an educational program that prepares registered nurses will take the NCLEX, the national nursing licensure examination prepared under the supervision of the National Council of State Boards of Nursing. NCLEX is taken after graduation and prior to practice as a registered nurse. The examination is given across the United States. Graduates submit their credentials to the state board of nursing in the state in which licensure is desired. Once the state board accepts the graduate's credentials, the graduate can schedule the examination. This examination ensures a basic level of safe registered nursing practice to the public. The examination follows a test plan formulated on four categories of client needs that registered nurses commonly encounter. The concepts of the nursing process, caring, communication, cultural awareness, documentation, self-care, and teaching/learning are integrated throughout the four major categories of client needs (Table F-1).

■ TOTAL NUMBER OF QUESTIONS ON NCLEX

Graduates may receive anywhere from 75 to 265 questions on the NCLEX examination during their testing session. Fifteen of the questions are questions that are being piloted to determine their validity for use in future NCLEX examinations. Students cannot determine whether they passed or failed the NCLEX examination from the number of questions they receive during their session. There is no time limit for each question, and the maximum time for the examination is 5 hours. A 10-minute break is mandatory after 2 hours of testing. An optional 10-minute break may be taken after another 90 minutes of testing.

TABLE F-1   NCLEX Test Plan: Client Needs

Client Needs Tested	Percent of Test Questions
Safe, effective care environment:	
Management of care	7-13%
Safety and infection control	5-11%
Physiologic integrity:	
Basic care and comfort	7-13%
Pharmacological and parenteral therapies	5-11%
Reduction of risk potential	12-18%
Physiological adaptation	12-18%
Psychosocial integrity:	
Coping and adaptation	5-11%
Psychosocial adaptation	5-11%
Health promotion and maintenance:	
Growth and development through the life span	7-13%
Prevention and early detection of disease	5-11%

Each test question has a test item and four possible answers. If the student answers the question correctly, a slightly more difficult item will follow, and the level of difficulty will increase with each item until the candidate misses an item. If the student misses an item, a slightly less difficult item will follow, and the level of difficulty will decrease with each item until the student has answered an item correctly. This process continues until the student has achieved a definite passing or definite failing score. The least number of questions a student can take to complete the exam is 75. Fifteen of these

TABLE F-2   Factors Associated with NCLEX Performance

- HESI Exit Exam
- Mosby Assesstest
- NLN Comprehensive Achievement test
- NLN achievement tests taken at end of each nursing course
- Verbal SAT score
- ACT score

- High school rank and GPA
- Undergraduate nursing program GPA
- GPA in science and nursing theory courses
- Competency in American English language
- Reasonable family responsibilities or demands
- Absence of emotional distress
- Critical thinking competency

questions will be pilot questions, and they will not count toward the student's score. The other 60 questions will determine the student's score on the NCLEX.

■ RISK FACTORS FOR NCLEX PERFORMANCE

Several factors have been identified as being associated with perform-ance on the NCLEX examination. Some of these factors are identified in Table F-2.

■ REVIEW BOOKS AND COURSES

In preparing to take the NCLEX, the new graduate may find it useful to review several of the many NCLEX review books on the market. These review books often include a review of nursing content, or sample test questions, or both. They frequently include computer software disks with test questions for review.The test questions may be arranged in the review book by clinical content area, or they may be presented in one or more comprehensive examinations covering all areas of the NCLEX. Listings of these review books are available at *www.amazon.com*. It is helpful to use several of these books and computer software when reviewing for the NCLEX.

NCLEX review courses are also available. Brochures advertising these pro-grams are often sent to schools and are available in many sites nationwide. The quality of these programs can vary, and students may want to ask former nursing graduates and faculty for recommendations.

■ THE NLN EXAMINATION AND THE HESI EXIT EXAM

Many nursing programs administer an examination to students at the completion of their nursing program. Two of these exams are the NLN Achievement test and the HESI Exit Exam. New graduates will want to review their performance on any of these exams because these results will help identify their weaknesses and help focus their review sessions.

Students who examine their feedback from the NLN examination or the HESI Exit Exam have important information that can help them focus their review for the NCLEX. A strategy for examining this feedback and organizing this review is outlined in the following section.

■ ORGANIZING YOUR REVIEW

In preparing for NCLEX, identify your strengths and weaknesses. If you have taken the NLN examination or the HESI Exit Exam, note any content strength and weakness areas. Additionally, note any nursing program course or clinical content areas in which you scored below a grade of B. Purchase one or more of the NCLEX review books. It is useful to review questions developed by different authors. Review content in the review books in any of your weak content areas.Take a comprehensive exam in the review book or on the computer software disk and analyze your performance. Try to answer as many questions correctly as you can. Be sure to actually practice taking the examinations. Do not just jump ahead to look at the section on correct answers and rationales before answering the questions if you want to improve your examination performance.

Next, once you have completed the comprehensive examination, review the answers and rationales for any weak content areas and take another comprehensive exam. Repeat this process until you are doing well in all clinical content areas and in all areas of the NCLEX examination plan.

Finally, do a general review of the top 10 patient diseases, medications, diagnostic tests, and nursing procedures in each major nursing content area, as well as defense mechanisms, communication tips, and growth and development. Practice visualization and relaxation techniques as needed. These strategies will assist you in conquering the three areas necessary for successful test taking—anxiety control, content review, and test question practice. Table F-3 will help organize your study.

■ WHEN TO STUDY

Identify your personal best time.Are you a day person? Are you a night person? Study when you are fresh. Arrange to study 1 or more hours daily. Use Table F-4 to organize your study if you have 1 month to go.

Students who use this technique should increase their confidence in their ability to do well on the NCLEX.

TABLE F-3　Preparation for the NCLEX Test

Name: _____

Strengths: _____

Weak content areas identified on NLN examination or HESI Exit Exam:
_____
_____
_____

Weak content areas identified by yourself or others during formal nursing education program (include content areas in which you scored below a grade of B in class or any factors from Table F-2):
_____
_____
_____

Weak content areas identified in any area of the NCLEX test plan, including the following:

　　Safe, effective care environment

　　Physiological integrity

　　Psychosocial integrity

　　Health promotion and maintenance

Weak content areas identified in any of the top 10 patient diagnoses in each of the following:

　　Adult health

　　Women's health

　　Mental health nursing

　　Children's health
　　　　(Consider the 10 top medications, diagnostic tools and tests, treatments and
　　　　procedures used for each of the ten diagnoses.)

Weak content areas identified in the following:

　　Therapeutic communication tools

　　Defense mechanisms

　　Growth and development

　　Other

TABLE F-4 Organizing Your NCLEX Study

Note your weaknesses identified in Table F-3.

Take a comprehensive exam from one of the review books and analyze your performance. Then, depending on this test performance and the weaknesses identified in Table F-3, your schedule could look like the following:

Day 1: Practice adult health test questions. Score the test, analyze your performance, and review test question rationales and content weaknesses.

Day 2: Practice women's health test questions. Repeat above process.

Day 3: Practice children's health test questions. Repeat above process.

Day 4: Practice mental health test questions. Repeat above process.

Day 5: Continue with other weak content areas. Continue this process until you are doing well in all areas of the test.

Glossary

Abandonment   Negligence in which a client is left in need without alternatives for treatment.

Acquaintance (or Date) Rape   Forcible rape or sexual battery that occurs by the victim's acquaintances or dates.

Adaptive Energy   Individual's ability to respond to a stressor.

Adaptive Potential   Capacity of the person to respond to stressors—to utilize resources to cope.

Adaptive Potential Assessment Model   Erickson and colleagues' model describing three states of coping potential: arousal, equilibrium, and impoverishment.

Addiction   Inability to abstain from drug use, accompanied by drug tolerance and withdrawal.

Adversity   Measure of the strength of a given stimulus for anxiety.

Aggravated Criminal Sexual Assault   Criminal sexual assault in which a weapon is used or displayed; the victim's life or someone else's is endangered or threatened; the perpetrator causes bodily harm to the victim; the assault occurs during the commission of another felony; or force is used to threaten or cause physical harm to the victim.

Aggregate   Population or defined group.

Agnosia   Loss of ability to recognize objects.

Agoraphobia   Fear of going out in public places.

Akathisia   Subjective sense of restlessness with a perceived need to pace or otherwise move continuously.

Akinesia   Reaction involving loss of movement.

Alcoholism   Compulsion to drink alcohol.

Alogia   Tendency to speak very little and use brief and seemingly empty phrases.

Amnesia   Loss of memory.

Anger Control Assistance   Nursing intervention aimed at facilitation of the expression of anger in an adaptive and nonviolent manner.

Anhedonia   Inability to find enjoyment in daily activities.

Animal-Assisted Therapy   Use of animals to provide attention, affection, diversion, and/or relaxation.

Anorexia Nervosa   Psychological eating disorder characterized by profound disturbance in body image, failure to maintain minimum weight, and obsession with weight, despite underweight status.

Antipsychotic Drugs   Major tranquilizers administered to control symptoms of psychosis.

Antisocial Personality Disorder
Behavior pattern characterized by violence, impulsiveness, dishonesty, carelessness, and irresponsibility.

Anxiety   State where a person has strong feelings of worry or dread, where the source is nonspecific or unknown.

Aphasia   Difficulty or inability to recall words.

Apraxia   Loss of motor function.

Arousal   Stress state in which an individual possesses coping resources.

Asperger's Syndrome   Condition characterized by combination of severe impairments in social interaction and highly repetitive patterns of interests and behaviors.

Asylum   Large public hospital of the eighteenth century that provided for treatment of the insane.

Autism   Developmental disorder in which children remain emotionally detached, engage in ritualistic behavior, and exhibit delay in acquiring language skills.

Autonomy   Individual's right to self-determination and independence.

Avoidant Personality Disorder
Behavior pattern characterized by social inhibition, feelings of inadequacy, and shyness.

Avolition   Lack of motivation for work or other goal-oriented activities.

Behaviorally Oriented Therapy
Process focused on helping an individual gain the tools needed to change behavior and feelings.

Beneficence   Belief that all treatments must be for the client's good.

Bipolar Depression   Mood disorder characterized by up-and-down swings.

Bipolar Disorder (BPD)   Mood disorder characterized by cyclic experiences with both mania and depression.

Blinded Clinical Trial   Study in which subjects do not know whether they are receiving an active treatment or a placebo.

Blood-Brain Barrier   Capillary barrier between blood and brain.

Borderline Personality Disorder
Disorder characterized by unstable interpersonal relationships and self-image, efforts to avoid being abandoned, and impulsive actions.

Breathing-Related Sleep Disorders
A group of disorders in which breathing during sleep stops for less than 10 seconds, occurring 20 or more times per hour and causing measurable blood deoxygenation.

Brief Dynamic Therapy   Short-term psychotherapy that focuses on resolving core conflicts that derive from personality and living situations.

Brown Report   A 1948 report authored by Esther Lucille Brown on the future of nursing. This report advised that psychiatric hospitals be used as agencies for affiliation in teaching of nurses.

Bulimia Nervosa   Psychological eating disorder characterized by fasting, binging, purging (by either self-induced vomiting or misuse of laxatives, diuretics, or enemas), and lack of extreme weight loss.

Burnout   Description for caregivers who find themselves unable to provide the quality of care that is desirable; characterized by depletion of energy, decreased ability to concentrate, and a sense of hopelessness.

Capitation   Funding mechanism in which all defined services for a specified period of time are provided for an agreed-on single payment.

Case-Control Study   Study comparing two groups: the cases (all members have the given disease or condition) and the controls (all members are free of the disease or condition).

Case Group *See* Experimental Group.

Case Management Constellation of services that includes screening, assessment, care planning, arranging for service delivery, monitoring, reassessment, evaluation, and discharge, for the purpose of ensuring continuity of care.

Cataplexy Sudden loss of muscle power at times of sudden emotion.

Catastrophic Reaction Severe overreaction out of proportion to the stimulus.

Catatonia Behavior disorder marked by a decrease in reactivity to the environment, sometimes reaching an extreme degree of complete unawareness.

Catharsis Experience of release that occurs when unconscious thoughts are brought into consciousness.

Child Abuse Any physical or mental injury, sexual abuse, exploitation, negligent treatment, or maltreatment of a child by a parent or caregiver.

Child Molestation Sexual involvement with a child, such as oral-genital contact, genital fondling and viewing, or masturbation in front of a child.

Child Pornography Sexually explicit reproduction of a child's image.

Choice Point Time in a person's life when previously successful activities are no longer solving disruptions in one's life patterns.

Chronic Grief Unresolved bereavement.

CINAHL The Cumulative Index of Nursing and Allied Health Literature; a Nursing-specific search tool for published literature.

Circadian Rhythm Biorhythm that determines human responses to the environment; refers to attention span in relation to the presence or absence of daylight.

Circular Communication Predictable pattern of communication and response between two people.

Civil Commitment Period of hospitalization requested by a mental health provider following an emergency hospitalization.

Clarification Technique in which an analyst points out a behavior pattern that is not recognized by the client.

Classification System of categorization that allows useful distinctions to be established.

Client-Centered Therapy Process focused on bringing out individual internal resources and understanding.

Closed Group Meeting with a defined number of participants that is not open to new members.

Code of Ethics Positive statements and guidelines of what persons should do.

Codependence Behaviors exhibited by significant others of a substance-abusing individual that serve to enable and protect the abuse at the exclusion of personal fulfillment and self-development.

Cognator Subsystem Higher brain functions that deal with information processing, judgment, emotion, and perception.

Cognition Process by which a person "knows the world" and interacts with it.

Cognitive-Behavior(al) Therapy Treatment approach aimed at helping a client identify stimuli that cause the client's anxiety, develop plans to respond to those stimuli in a nonanxious manner, and problem-solve when unanticipated anxiety-provoking situations arise.

Cognitive Therapy Short-term psychotherapy that focuses on removing symptoms by identifying and correcting perceptual biases in client's thinking and correcting unrecognized assumptions.

Cohort Study *See* Longitudinal Study.

Community Crisis Threat of proportion to affect an entire group of people.

Community Health Nursing Synthesis of nursing and public health practice to promote, maintain, and conserve the health of population aggregates in the community.

Community Mental Health Synthesis of community nursing and public health practice to promote, maintain, and conserve the health of population aggregates in the community, with particular emphasis on mental health.

Community Support System (CSS) Organized network of people committed to helping persons with severe mental illness meet their needs and move toward independence.

Competency to Stand Trial Judgment that an individual is able to understand the nature of legal proceedings and is able to tell his or her own story to an attorney and the court.

Complementary Modalities Those modalities being used as an adjunct to medical care and psychiatric treatment that are thought to have effects on stress, sleep disturbance, anxiety, and/or other emotions.

Compulsion Repetitive behavior or act, the goal of which is to prevent or reduce anxiety or distress.

Computerized Tomography A scan that uses conventional X-rays to form an image that is an actual reconstruction from hundreds of X-rays taken from various angles.

Concept Basic building block of theory; abstraction of reality.

Concept Map A diagrammatic representation of organized knowledge. In nursing care, a diagrammatic representation of the nursing process, illustrating the relationships between and among issues and characteristics that emerge from assessment data.

Conceptual Framework Group of concepts that are linked together to provide a way of organizing or viewing something.

Conduct Disorder Disorder in which children show a pattern of cruelty and disrespect for the rights of others.

Confabulation Intentional efforts to cover up memory losses or gaps.

Confrontation Technique in which an analyst challenges a client's behavior or thought, with the goal of provoking a reaction and overcoming an emotional barrier to change.

Confusion Multidimensional phenomenon incorporating changes in both cognition and behavior.

Conservative-Withdrawal State Psychological response to stress; stage of exhaustion.

Conservator Person appointed to handle the estate of another person who is judged incompetent.

Continuous Cycling Recurrent movement from mania to depression without an intervening normal period.

Control Group Persons receiving no treatment or being free of a given condition or disease under study.

Controlled Clinical Trial Evaluation in which neither the clients nor their caregivers are allowed to know exactly what treatment is being given.

Conversion Disorder Condition in which an individual exhibits physical symptoms that cannot be explained by any medical or neurological conditions.

Cortex The part of the brain consisting of the four lobes: frontal, temporal, parietal, and occipital.

Craving Strong, overpowering urge for drugs felt by an individual who abuses or is dependent on drugs.

Created Environment Mobilization of all system variables.

Criminal Sexual Assault Genital, anal, or oral penetration by a part of the perpetrator's body or by an object using force or without the victim's consent.

Crisis   Stressor or life challenge that requires an individual to adjust to the unexpected and to adapt to an unpredicted situation or event.

Cultural Blindness   Attempt to treat all persons fairly by ignoring differences and acting as though differences do not exist; misguided attempt to achieve "fairness" by ignoring real cultural differences.

Cultural Crisis   Situation of shock resulting from an individual's adaptation to a new culture or return to a previously experienced culture; also known as culture shock.

Cultural Facilitator/Broker   Person who can interpret the language, culture, and health care culture of another as a means to bridging the communication barriers between people from different cultures.

Culture   Values, beliefs, norms, and lifeways that are learned and shared within a particular group.

Culture Care   Facets of culture that deal with individual and group health and well-being, including efforts to improve on the human condition or to deal with illness, handicaps, or death.

Culture Care Accommodation/Negotiation   Nursing actions and decisions that involve reshaping the way in which care values are enacted so the actions will better support well-being, dealing with handicaps, recovering from illness, or facing death.

Culture Care Preservation/Maintenance   Nursing actions and decisions that help people of a cultural group keep or preserve those care values that are applicable to the current situation to maintain well-being, deal with handicaps, recover from illness, or face death.

Culture Care Repatterning/Restructuring   Nursing actions and decisions

that involve change in culturally based care practices.

Culture Shock   State in which a person is overwhelmed or even immobilized by cultural differences in expectations, communication, and general habits between an individual's culture of origin and a new culture to which the individual is trying to assimilate. (*See* also Cultural Crisis)

Cyclothymic Pattern   Cycle of an individual's mood changing back and forth between hypomanic and melancholic states.

Defense Mechanisms   Unconscious responses used by individuals to protect themselves from internal conflict and external stress.

Deinstitutionalization   Movement of clients and mental health services from state mental hospitals into community settings.

Delayed Grief   Bereavement that is not accomplished at the time of the loss and remains with the individual.

Delirium   Acute change in a person's level of consciousness and cognition that develops during a short period.

Delusion   False belief that misrepresents either perceptions or experiences.

Dementia   Gradual onset of multiple cognitive changes in memory, abstract thinking, judgment, and perception that often results in a progressive decline in intellectual functioning and decreased capacity to perform daily activities.

Deontology   Theory founded on human duties to others and the principles on which these duties are based.

Deoxyribonucleic Acid (DNA)   A molecule that carries a genetic code in its sequence of bases.

Dependent Personality Disorder Behavior pattern characterized by clinging and submissiveness.

Depersonalization   Persistent or recurrent feelings of being separated from one's normal mental fuctions or feeling as if one is outside one's body.

Depression   State wherein an individual experiences a profound sadness.

Derailment   Speech that gets off the point or subject.

Descriptive Study   Survey to determine the incidence and prevalence of a disease or condition.

Diencephalon   The part of the brain consisting of two major structures: the thalamus and the hypothalamus.

Differentiation   Process of unfolding, growth, and maturation, leading to a balance between emotional and intellectual components.

Disability   Impairment in one or more important areas of functioning.

Dissociative Disorders   Disorders characterized by a disruption in the usually integrated functions of consciousness, memory, identity, or perception.

Dissociative Identity Disorder   The condition of possessing two or more distinct identities, at least two of which periodically take control of the individual's behavior.

Distress   Negative response to stimuli that are perceived as threatening.

Double-Blinded Trial   Study in which neither subjects nor persons evaluating the outcome know whether subjects are receiving treatment or a placebo.

Drug Dependence   Condition occurring when individuals exhibit a set of behaviors associated with inability to control use of a drug.

Drug Use   Any taking of a drug.

DSM-IV-TR   *Diagnostic and Statistical Manual, Fourth edition-Text Revision;* classification system for mental disorders.

Dyssomnia   Condition where there is an abnormality in the amount, quality, or timing of sleep.

Dysthymia   Condition of feeling sad or depressed. Persistent state of sadness.

Dystonia   Sustained, involuntary muscle spasms.

Echolalia   An involuntary, parrotlike repetition of words spoken by others.

Ecomap   Graphic depiction of family members' interactions with systems outside the family.

Ego   Conscious mind governed by the reality principle; controls the impulses of the id.

Electroconvulsive Therapy (ECT) Passage of an electrical stimulus to the brain to produce a seizure.

Emergency Hospitalization   Power of states to detain a person in an emergency situation for a limited time until further evaluation and court proceedings can occur.

Emotional Cutoff   Children's efforts to distance themselves from their families in order to achieve independence; any family member's efforts to distance self from family and others to reduce anxiety.

Endemic   Descriptor for a disease or condition that is constantly or regularly found in the population.

Energy-Based Modalities   Techniques for healing grounded in the notion of the human energy field.

Epidemic   Descriptor for a disease or condition that spreads or circulates within a population.

Epidemiology   Study of the causes and distribution of injuries and diseases in a population.

Equilibrium   State of balance following a stress state.

Ethics   Branch of philosophy that considers how behavioral principles guiding human interactions can be analyzed and set.

Ethnicity Identification with a socially, culturally, and politically constructed group that holds a common set of characteristics not shared by others with whom its members come in contact.

Ethnocentrism Perception that one's worldview is the only acceptable truth and that the beliefs, values, and behaviors sanctioned by one's culture are superior to all others.

Euthanasia Act of killing or permitting a death for reasons of mercy.

Exaggerated Grief Bereavement that is overwhelming.

Exhibitionism Exposing one's genitals to a stranger.

Experience-Oriented Therapy Process focusing on the client's experiences as an agent for producing change.

Experimental Group Persons receiving treatment or having a given condition or disease under study; also known as Case Group.

External Environment Forces, factors, and influences that occur outside the boundaries of a system.

Extrapersonal Stressor Stimuli from a great distance outside the system boundary.

Factitious Disorder Condition marked by physical or psychological symptoms that are intentionally and knowingly produced by an individual in order to gain attention; also known as Munchausen's syndrome.

Family Social system composed of two or more persons who coexist within the context of some expectations of reciprocal affection, mutual responsibility, and temporal duration.

Family Attachment Diagram Representation of the reciprocal nature and quality of the affectional ties between family members.

Family Projection Process Situation in which adult family members deal with their own anxiety by projecting the anxiety onto a child.

Fear State wherein a person feels a strong sense of dread focused on a specific object or event.

Feedback Response of a receiver of a message to the communicator.

Fetishism Sexual arousal occurring from contact with a nonliving object, often an article of clothing.

Fidelity Individual's obligation to honor commitments and contracts.

Fight-Flight Response Psychological response to stress; state of high anxiety and energy.

Financial Abuse Theft or conversion of money or anything of value belonging to the elderly by their relatives or caregivers.

Fixation Preoccupation with pleasures associated with a previous developmental stage.

Flattened Affect Loss of expressiveness.

Folk System Culturally based acts that respond to apparent or anticipated needs related to living, health, well-being, handicaps, or death.

Forcible Rape Forced intercourse or penetration of a body orifice by a penis or other object by a perpetrator.

Foreclosure One of four identity statuses; refers to the adolescent's lack of thoroughly exploring alternatives before making a commitment to an adult identity.

Frotteurism Recurrent sexual touching of a nonconsenting individual, usually a stranger and usually in a crowded public place.

Fugue Sudden unexpected travel away from home or normal environment, usually associated with confusion about past identity.

Gang Rape   Sexual acts that proximate in time by multiple perpetrators who are either acquaintances of or strangers to the victim.

Gender Dysphoria   Condition existing when an individual has a strong desire to live as the opposite sex.

Gender Identity   An individual's subjective feeling associated with being male or female.

Gender Identity Disorder   Condition in which an individual feels him- or herself to be a member of the opposite sex and desires gender change.

Gender Role   Learned expressions of femaleness and maleness; public recognition of one's gender assignment as male or female and the individual's expression of appropriate social behaviors related to that assignment.

General Adaptation Syndrome   Specific, predictable, physiological response to stress involving an alarm reaction, a resistance stage, and an exhaustion stage.

Generalized Anxiety Disorder Psychiatric illness characterized by excessive anxiety or dread.

Genetic Marker   Identifiable patterns of DNA structure that can be readily confirmed by laboratory analysis.

Genogram   Graphic depiction of a family tree that records information over at least three generations.

Genome   Entire complement of heritable information.

Grandiose Delusion   Perception of importance, special powers, or religious significance that is not in line with reality.

Gradiosity   An inflated appraisal of one's worth, knowledge, power, or importance, often including delusional thinking.

Grief   Healthy expression of bereavement.

Group   Collection of persons who come together in some way that makes them interdependent.

Group Content   Specific problems, topics, or conditions addressed by a group.

Group Dynamics   Underlying forces working to produce behavior patterns in groups.

Group Leader/Facilitator   Person who invites or selects group members and identifies the purpose and goals of the group.

Group Process   Interaction (verbal and nonverbal) between and among group members.

Guided Imagery   An unconditional process in which the practitioner leads the subject with specific words, suggestions, symbols, or images to elicit a positive response.

Half-Life   Time for plasma concentrations of a drug to decrease to half of an initial value.

Hallucination   Sensory experiences not perceptible to other nonpsychotic individuals.

Healing Touch   Systematic approach to healing using several energy interventions that incorporate a variety of therapeutic maneuvers.

Helicy   The movement of human development toward increasing diversity and complexity.

HIPAA   The Health Insurance Portability and Accountability Act; federal legislation protecting the privacy of medical records.

Histrionic Personality Disorder   Behavior pattern characterized by excesses of emotional expression and a desire to be the center of attention.

Home Health Nursing   Delivery of health services in the home under the direction of a health care agency.

Homelessness   Condition of being without shelter or a permanent place to live.

Hypnosis   Assisting the client to an altered state of consciousness to create an awareness and a directed-focus experience.

Hypoactive Sexual Desire Disorder   Significant distress or disturbance in interpersonal relationships when the sexual desire is truly less than would be normal for an individual.

Hypochondriasis   Condition marked by preoccupation with fear of having a serious disease, based on misinterpretation of bodily symptoms or functions.

Hypomania   Mild form of mania (elevated mood) that lasts for at least 4 days.

Hypothalamus   A central brain structure that is primarily involved with the autonomic nervous system and the endocrine system and that plays a role in the nervous mechanisms underlying moods and motivational states.

ICD   *International Classification of Diseases;* a comprehensive listing of clinical diagnoses, each associated with a unique numerical code.

ICNP   The International Classification of Nursing Practice.

Id   Unconscious mind; the reservoir of psychic energy or libido.

Identity Achievement   One of the four identity statuses in which an adolescent makes a commitment to an adult identity after a period of exploring alternatives.

Identity Diffusion   One of the four identity statuses in which an adolescent avoids making a full commitment to an adult identity and does not reach his or her potential; often associated with restricted emotional expression or detachment from others.

Identity Formation   An adolescent's process of finding a unique place within the larger society, beyond the boundaries of the family.

Identity Status   Style used by an adolescent in resolving issues of adult identity.

Impoverishment   Stress state in which an individual's coping resources are depleted.

Incarcerated   Condition of being in jail or other correctional institution.

Incest   Sexual relations between children and blood relatives or surrogate family members.

Incidence   Number of new cases of an illness, condition, or injury that begin within a certain time period.

Incoherence   Speech that is not logically connected.

Incompetence   State of an individual with a mental disorder that causes inability to make judgments and renders the person unable to handle his or her own affairs.

Insight-Oriented Therapy   Process focusing on helping an individual gain understanding of feelings and behaviors.

Insomnia   Sleep disorder characterized by difficulty in initiating or maintaining sleep.

Integrality   The energy fields of the human being and of the environment are each part of the other's.

Intentionality   Consciousness and awareness directed mentally toward an object and involving expectation, belief, action, desire, and the unconscious.

Internal Environment   Forces, factors, and influences that occur completely within the boundaries of a system.

Interpersonal Stressor   Stimuli from outside the system boundary but proximal to the system.

Interpersonal Therapy   Process of gaining insight based on the recognition that psychological distress may occur in conjunction with disturbed human relationships.

Interpretation Technique in which an analyst offers an explanation of a client's unconscious behavior processes.

Interrater Agreement Accord on diagnosis between individuals evaluating the same condition.

Interrater Reliability Accord on diagnosis between different evaluators on the same examination.

Interventive Questions Circular questions used to uncover relationships and connections between individuals, events, ideas, and beliefs.

Intimate Partner Violence (Often referred to as spousal/partner abuse or battering syndrome.) Intentional violent or controlling behavior by a person who is or has been intimate with the victim(s) and may or may not reside in the same household.

Intrapersonal Stressor Stimuli from within the system boundary.

Intrarater Reliability Accord on diagnosis on different examinations by the same evaluator.

Justice Principle ensuring fairness, equity, and honesty in decisions.

Least Restrictive Alternative Legal principle requiring that clients be treated with the least amount of constraint of liberty consistent with their safety.

Light Therapy (Phototherapy) Provision of artificial indoor lighting, 5 to 10 times brighter than ordinary lighting, to the environment of a person with Seasonal Affective Disorder (SAD).

Longitudinal Study Population-based study conducted over a period of time, typically years; also known as Cohort Study.

Magnetic Resonance Imaging An imaging technique that uses no X-rays. The image is produced through use of a magnetic field, radio frequencies, and computerized reconstructions.

Malingering Fabrication of symptoms with the intent of achieving some objective goal.

Malpractice Negligence in the medical field that results in harm.

Managed Care Prepaid health plan in which an identified intermediary is given authority to manage the means and the source from which the client may obtain services.

Mania Mood disorder characterized by an elevated, expansive, or irritable mood.

Manic Episode Distinct period of abnormally and persistently elevated, expansive, or irritable mood, lasting at least 1 week.

Marital Therapy Short-term psychotherapy that attempts to resolve problems that occur within a marriage.

Masked Grief Bereavement that is hidden by either a physical symptom or a maladaptive behavior; the individual is unaware of the connection to the grief or loss.

Massage Stimulation of the skin and underlying tissues for the purposes of increasing circulation and inducing a relaxation response.

Maturational Crisis Stage in an individual's life requiring adjustment or adaptation to new responsibilities or life patterns.

Mental Disorder Behavior or psychological syndrome or pattern associated with distress or disability or increased risk of suffering, death, pain, or loss of freedom.

Mental Health State in which a person has knowledge of self, meets basic needs, assumes responsibility for behavior and self-growth, integrates thoughts and feelings with actions, resolves conflicts, maintains relationships, respects others, communicates directly, and adapts to change in the environment.

Mental Illness   State in which an individual shows deficits in functioning, cannot view self clearly or has a distorted image of self, is unable to maintain personal relationships, and cannot adapt to the environment.

Mental Injury   Harm to a child's psychological or intellectual functioning; manifested as severe anxiety, depression, withdrawal or outward aggressive behavior, or a combination of these behaviors.

Meta-Analysis   Statistical analysis that combines the results of several separate clinical studies.

Mind Modulation   Processes by which thoughts, feelings, attitudes, and emotions are converted by the brain into neurohormonal messenger molecules.

M'Naghten Test   Legal definition of lack of guilt of a crime by virtue of insanity.

Modeling   Assessment with the goal of understanding the client's world from the client's perspective.

Mood Disorder   Pattern of mood episodes that results in difficulty functioning in family, work, and social affairs.

Mood Episode   Experience of a strong emotion of depression, mania, or a mixture of both for a period of at least 2 weeks.

Moratorium   One of the four identity statuses in which an individual delays making a decision about adult identity while exploring various alternatives during adolescence.

Multigenerational Transmission Process   Situation in which patterns of dealing with anxiety are passed from one generation to the next.

Munchausen's Syndrome   Another term for Factitious Disorder.

Munchausen's Syndrome by Proxy
Form of child abuse marked by a caregiver falsely giving reports of a child's illness that result in unnecessary medical investigations or treatments.

Music Therapy   Use of specific kinds of music and its ability to affect changes in behavior, emotions, and physiology.

Mutuality   Client involvement in the therapeutic relationship.

NANDA   NANDA International prepared a taxonomy of nursing diagnoses, which are statements of the phenomena of concern to nurses.

Narcissistic Personality Disorder
Behavior pattern characterized in part by lack of empathy for others and a grandiose sense of self-importance.

Narcolepsy   Sleep disorder characterized by frequent irresistible urges for sleep, hallucinatory dreamlike states, and episodes of cataplexy.

National Mental Health Act   Provided federal funds for research and education in all areas of psychiatric care. Act was passed in 1946. Established NIMH.

Negligence   Behaving in a way in which a prudent individual would not have behaved or failing to use the diligence and care expected of a reasonable individual in similar circumstances.

Negligent Treatment   Failure of a parent or caregiver to provide, for reasons other than poverty, adequate food, clothing, shelter, or medical care, which may lead to serious endangerment of the physical health of the child.

Neologistic Word   Invented word, often used by persons suffering from schizophrenia.

Neuroleptic Malignant Syndrome
Disorder associated with sudden fever, rigidity, tachycardia, hypertension, and decreased levels of consciousness.

Neurotransmitter A chemical messenger that permits the movement of ions and chemicals across synapses.

NIC *Nursing Interventions Classification;* outlines list of nursing interventions designed to identify activities that nurses perform to assist client status or behavior.

Nightmare Exceedingly vivid dream from which the sleeper wakens in fear, often sweating and with heart racing, and is able to recall the dream.

NIMBY Syndrome Literally, "not in my backyard." Condition of persons or groups who state support for services for the homeless or underprivileged groups but who refuse to allow such services in their own neighborhoods.

NMDS Nursing Minimum Data Set; grouping that identifies the minimum information necessary to meet information demands of nursing practice.

Nonmaleficence Belief that care providers must do no harm.

Nonverbal Communication Messages sent by means other than oral or written.

Normal Sexual Behavior Any sexual act that is consensual, lacks force, is mutually satisfying to both partners, and is conducted in private. [For adults]

Normative Ethics Guidelines and procedures useful in establishing moral decisions and actions.

Norms Learned behaviors that are perceived to be appropriate or inappropriate in a culture.

Nuclear Family Emotional System Process by which a family manages anxiety.

Nurse Agency Nursing activities required to compensate for the client's inability to meet his own self-care needs (Orem's theory).

Nursing Agency Characteristic that allows nurses to act for others in meeting therapeutic self-care demands.

Nursing Care Plan A method of documenting the steps of the nursing process that includes a statement related to each step of the process: assessment, diagnosis, outcomes identification, planning/interventions, and evaluation.

Nursing System The design of care based on the type of self-care deficit.

Obsession Recurrent thought, image, or impulse that is experienced as intrusive and inappropriate and that causes marked anxiety or distress.

Obsessive-Compulsive Personality Disorder Behavior pattern characterized by preoccupation with order, cleanliness, control, and perfectionism.

Oculogyric Crisis Reaction in which extraocular muscle spasm forces the eyes into a fixed, usually upward gaze.

Open Group Meeting in which participants are free to come and go, depending on their individual needs.

Oppositional Defiant Disorder Condition characterized by a consistent pattern of rejecting authority.

Orientation The phase of the nurse-patient relationship in which they come to know each other and begin to identify the patient's needs.

Orientation Phase First stage of a relationship, during which the nurse and client get to know one another, establish trust, and outline goals and boundaries.

Panic Disorder Psychiatric illness characterized by discrete episodes of intense anxiety (panic attacks) that begin abruptly and peak within 10 minutes.

Paranoid Personality Disorder Behavior pattern characterized by persistent yet unfounded fear of exploitation or harm by others.

Paraphilia Disorder of sexual interest, arousal, and orgasm.

Parasomnia Condition in which the person suffers from profoundly disturbed sleep, most commonly nightmares, sleep terrors, or sleepwalking.

Parasympathetic System Response Nervous system response that works in opposition to the sympathetic nervous system, bringing about a decrease in heart and respiratory rates, dilation of peripheral blood vessels, muscle relaxation, lowered blood pressure, and increased flow of endorphins.

Passive-Aggressive Personality Disorder Behavior pattern characterized by pervasive negativity with passive resistance to social/occupational demands, procrastination, and stubbornness.

Passive Physical Abuse (or Negligence) Conduct that is careless and a breach of duty that results in injury to the person or is a violation of rights; includes the withholding of medication, medical treatment, food, and personal care necessary for the well-being of the elderly person.

Pedophilia Sexual interests directed primarily or exclusively toward children.

Persecutory Delusion Paranoid perception that others are "out to get me."

Personality Habitual patterns and qualities of behavior expressed by physical and mental activities and attitudes; the distinctive individual qualities of a person.

Personality Disorder Pervasive and inflexible pattern of behavior demonstrating unhealthy characteristics that limit the individual's ability to function in society.

Personality Traits Qualities of behavior that make a person unique.

Phobia Persistent fear of a specific object or situation.

Physical Abuse Conduct of violence that results in bodily harm or mental stress; includes a spectrum of violence ranging from assault to murder.

Physical Injury Lacerations, fractured bones, burns, internal injuries, severe bruising, or serious bodily harm.

Physical Restraint Use of an apparatus that significantly inhibits mobility.

Placebo Treatment that has no intended effect on the expected outcome of a trial.

Population Aggregate of persons in the community who share a common characteristic, such as age or diagnosis.

Positron Emission Tomography (PET) A scan that requires the injection of a radioactive contrast that permits visualization of precise areas of the brain where functions like blood flow can be observed.

Post-Traumatic Stress Disorder Anxiety disorder resulting from a frightening event such as a crime, accident, or battle.

Power Influences each family member has on the family processes and functioning.

Presence Activity of being physically present with another person that begins with the nurse's genuine commitment to caring and nurturing the potential of the client.

Prevalence Number of persons in a population who are living with a disease or disorder at any time; includes both new and old cases.

Primary Hypersomnia Severe daytime sleepiness despite normal nighttime sleep patterns that interferes with daily activities; a condition that cannot be explained by any other sleep, medical, or pharmacological cause.

Primary Insomnia Condition in which an individual can fall asleep easily and remain asleep for several hours but does not feel rested on waking.

Primary Prevention Activities directed at reducing the incidence of mental disorder within a population.

Probate Proceedings Judicial hearing to determine the competence of an individual to manage personal affairs.

Process Recording Verbatim account of a communication, with interpretation of techniques used and their effectiveness.

Professional System Acts based on formal preparation for dealing with health, illness, and wellness.

Program for Assertive Community Treatment (PACT) Model providing a full range of medical, psychosocial, and rehabilitation services by a community-based, multi-disciplinary team.

Prospective Payment System Reimbursement mechanism based on predetermined payment for a specific period or diagnosis.

Psychiatric Consultation-Liaison Nursing Practice concerned with the study, diagnosis, treatment, and prevention of psychiatric illness in the physically ill and of psychological factors affecting physical conditions.

Psychiatric Mental Health Advanced Practice Registered Nurse A licensed nurse educationally certified at the masters or doctoral level and nationally certified as a clinical specialist in psychiatric and mental health nursing.

Psychiatric Mental Health Nurse A licensed nurse who has passed a certification exam and is thereby certified within a specialty.

Psychoanalysis Treatment focused on uncovering unconscious memories and processes.

Psychodynamic Therapy Brief process based on psychoanalytic principles, with the goal of improved functioning rather than personality reconstruction.

Psychological Abuse Simple name calling and verbal assaults in a protracted and systematic effort to dehumanize the victim, sometimes with the goal of driving the victim to insanity or suicide; usually exists in combination with one or more other abuses.

Psychological Development Continuum of milestones from infancy through adulthood showing evolution of personal history.

Psychosis State in which an individual has lost the ability to recognize reality.

Psychotherapy Treatment of mental or emotional disorders through psychological rather than physical methods.

Psychotic Mental state involving the loss of rational thought and/or loss of ability to accurately interpret the environment.

Public Health Nursing Field of nursing that addresses the social, economic, and environmental conditions that influence health.

PubMed A public-domain search tool of published medical literature sponsored by the National Library of Medicine (NLM).

Quasi-Experimental Study Analytical study in which a population is studied before and after a given event; usually includes both a case and a control set.

Rape Act of sexual intercourse in which the person does not give consent; accomplished against a person's will by means of force or fear of immediate and unlawful bodily injury or threatening to retaliate in the future against the victim or other person.

Rapid Cycling Four or more episodes of mania in a year.

Reactive Depression Adjustment disorder with depressed mood.

Referential Delusion Perception that common events refer specifically to the individual.

Regression Reversion to pleasures of a previous developmental stage.

Regulator Subsystem Human processes related to the autonomic nervous system and involving chemical, neural, and endocrine responses.

Relativistic Thinking Process of understanding the contextual nature of the world from multiple perspectives.

Relaxation A psychophysiological state characterized by parasympathetic dominance involving multiple visceral and somatic symptoms, including the absence of physical, mental, and emotional tension.

Reliability Measurement of reproducibility of a testing instrument.

Repression Process in which painful memories, thoughts, or experiences are actively kept out of conscious awareness.

Resonancy The movement of human energy wave patterns from low and slow to high and fast.

Risk Factors Traits that predispose an individual to a disease.

Role-Modeling Developing an individualized plan of care based on the client's world model.

Schizoaffective Disorder Condition characterized by elements of schizophrenia and manic-depressive disorder.

Schizoid Personality Disorder Behavior pattern characterized by lack of emotion and close friendships and detachment from persons and events in the immediate environment.

Schizophrenia Mental disorder characterized by disordered thoughts, hallucinations, and delusions.

Schizotypal Personality Disorder Behavior pattern characterized by inability to form close relations and a pattern of cognitive and perceptual distortions and eccentricities.

Search Engines Internet tools that allow the user to find Web sites based on words entered into the engines.

Seclusion State of a client being put in an isolated room or cell.

Secondary Prevention Activities directed at reducing the prevalence of mental disorders by shortening the duration of a sufficient number of established cases.

Self-Awareness Perception of oneself in relation to others and relative to society's expectations.

Self-Care Activities that humans perform for themselves to maintain life, to function, and to develop.

Self-Care Agency Ability to perform self-care in light of gender, age, socioeconomic status, developmental level, health, family, environment, living patterns, and availability of resources.

Self-Care Deficit State that occurs when an individual's therapeutic self-care demand is greater than the capacity to meet that demand.

Self-Efficacy Ability to organize and manage individual responses to the demands of the environment.

Self-Help Group Persons coming together who are facing a common difficulty.

Separation Anxiety Anxiety and fear experienced by a child when forced to separate from his/her parents.

Serotonergic Syndrome Drug reaction involving agitation, sweating, rigidity, fever, hyperreflexia, tachycardia, and hypotension.

Sexual Abuse (Child) Employment, use, persuasion, inducement, enticement, or coercion of a child to engage in, or assist another person to engage in sexually implicit conduct; includes rape, molestation, prostitution, or other forms of sexual exploitation of children or incest with children.

Sexual Abuse (Elder) Threat of sexual assault or actual sexual battery, rape, incest, sodomy, oral copulation, penetration of genital or anal opening by a foreign object, coerced nudity, and sexually explicit photographing.

Sexual Battery Activity of a person touching an intimate part (sexual organs, groin, buttocks, breast) of another person, if that touching is against the will of the person touched and is for the purpose of sexual arousal, gratification, or abuse.

Sexual Dysfunction Condition existing when a person experiences a change with any aspect of sexuality that is viewed as unsatisfying, unrewarding, or inadequate.

Sexual Exploitation Child pornography, sexually explicit reproduction of a child's image, or child prostitution.

Sexual Masochism Disorder characterized by sexual excitement resulting from fantasies or behaviors about being the recipient of physical abuse or humiliation.

Sexual Sadism Disorder characterized by sexual excitement resulting from persistent fantasies or behaviors involving infliction of suffering on others.

Sexually Explicit Conduct Actual or simulated sexual intercourse, bestiality, masturbation, lascivious exhibition of the genitals of a person or animal, or sadistic or masochistic abuse.

Sibling Position Birth order of children.

Situational Crisis Event that poses a threat or challenge to an individual.

Sleep Hygiene Specific activities that assist many persons to achieve restful sleep.

Sleep Latency Time it takes to fall asleep.

Sleep Paralysis Sensation of being unable to move, speak, or breathe during sleep.

Sleep Terrors Parasomnia in which there is *no recall* of the sleep-related event.

Sleepwalking Pattern of sleep behavior usually including getting out of bed, walking around in the bedroom, or on occasion outside of the bedroom, and then returning to bed.

SNOMED Systematized Nomenclature of Medicine; coding system that includes nursing diagnoses, nursing interventions, multiple axes that identify causative factors of illness, and related functional deficits and social factors.

Social Competence Degree to which significant others rate an individual as successful at performing expected social tasks.

Social Phobia Social anxiety, fear of being embarrassed in social settings.

Societal Regression Process of reversion in which anxiety leads to emotionally based decision making.

Somatic Therapies Interventions used in the management of psychiatric symptoms, for example, use of seclusion or physical restraints in control of anger.

Somatization Disorder Somatoform disorder in which there are multiple physical complaints without an apparent physiological cause.

Somatoform Disorder Psychiatric condition manifested in physical rather than psychological symptoms.

Spousal Rape Sexual intercourse against the victim's will by the spouse; accompanied by force, fear of bodily harm, or future retaliation.

Statutory Rape Sexual activity with a person under the age of consent (in most states, under 16 years of age) and considered to have occurred despite the apparent willingness of the underage person.

Stereotyping Assumption that people sharing certain characteristics will think and act similarly.

Stranger Rape Aggravated criminal sexual assault, forcible rape, or sexual battery that is committed against a victim by persons not acquainted with the victim.

Stress Stimulus that an individual perceives as challenging or harmful.

Substance Abuse Maladaptive pattern of use of a drug in situations of real or potential harm.

Suggestion Psychoanalytic technique in which the analyst interprets the client's thoughts, actions, or dreams.

Suicidal Ideation Thoughts of taking one's life.

Suicide Purposefully taking one's own life.

Suicide Potential Person's risk level for completing a suicide.

Suicide Survivor Friend or family member of an individual who dies from suicide.

Superego Conscious mind, governed by conscience and ego ideal.

Supportive-Educative Role Nursing activities that focus on enhancing the client's ability both to carry on effectively without nursing support and to rise above the feelings of depression (Orem's Theory).

Supportive Group Persons coming together to offer support, education, socialization, and/or recreation.

Switch Process Mood changes between mania and depression.

Sympathetic System Response Nervous system responses to stress that include increased heart rate, breathing, and blood pressure; constriction of peripheral blood vessels; muscle tension; gastric hyperacidity; release of adrenaline; and formation of cortisol.

Synapse Structure formed in which axons and dendrites come together.

Tangentiality Speech marked by failure to reach a goal or stick to the original point.

Tarasoff Duty to Warn Legal obligation of health care professionals to advise potential victims of violence so that the potential victim may seek protection.

Tardive Dyskinesia Neurological disorder characterized by involuntary movements, usually of the tongue and lips.

Termination The final phase of the nurse-patient relationship in which the relationship is ended after the patient's needs have been met.

Tertiary Prevention Activities directed at reducing the residual defects that are associated with mental disorders.

Thalamus An exceptionally important brain region that serves to relay a wide range of sensory inputs to the cerebral cortex; it is also a critical structure for maintaining consciousness.

Theory A set of interrelated concepts that provide testable relationships and direction or prediction.

Therapeutic Communication Purposeful use of dialogue to bring about the client's insight, control of symptoms, and healing. Communication that builds a trusting relationship.

Therapeutic Imagery The ability to take one's natural thought processes and direct those thoughts in a creative way, potentiating a positive outcome.

Therapeutic Massage Extension of massage techniques, involving deep tissue and advanced massage techniques.

Therapeutic Self-Care Demand Activities needed to meet self-care requisites to fulfill 21self-care agency.

Therapeutic Touch (TT) Five-step process of touch that involves centering; assessing the client's energy field; smoothing, or ''unruffling,'' the field; modulating or transferring energy; and knowing when to stop.

Therapeutic Window Time for peak effectiveness of a drug.

Therapy Group   Persons coming together to receive psychotherapy.

Tolerance   Acquired resistance to the effects of a drug.

Trait Anxiety   Personality characteristic reflecting susceptibility to anxiety.

Transvestic Fetishism   Cross-dressing or fantasies about cross-dressing.

Triangulation   Relational pattern among three members.

UMLS   Unified Medical Language System: thesaurus of all terms included in existing taxonomies.

Unipolar Depression   Disorder in which mood swings are always in one direction, toward depression.

Utilitarianism   Theory based on the principle that an ethical decision serves to produce the greatest good for the greatest number of persons.

Validity   Measurement of accuracy of a testing instrument.

Values   Learned beliefs about what is held to be good or bad in a culture.

Victim Consciousness   Belief that one is at the mercy of circumstances beyond one's control.

Violation of Rights   Abuse that occurs when the inalienable rights provided by the U.S. Constitution and federal statutes are violated by a family member or caregiver; includes such rights as not to have one's property taken without due process, the right to adequate appropriate medical treatment, and the right to freedom of assembly, speech, and religion.

Voyeurism   Observing or fantasizing about observing others disrobing, naked, or involved in sexual activity.

Withdrawal   Condition occurring when cessation of drug use results in a drug-specific set of symptoms that would be relieved by additional doses of the drug.

Word Salad   Speech marked by a group of disconnected words.

Working Phase   The phase of the nurse-patient relationship in which the nurse and patient work together to meet the patient's needs.

Code Legend

NP	**Phases of the Nursing Process**	Ph/7	Reduction of Risk Potential
As	Assessment	Ph/8	Physiological Adaptation
An	Analysis		
Pl	Planning	**CL**	**Cognitive Level**
Im	Implementation	K	Knowledge
Ev	Evaluation	Co	Comprehension
		Ap	Application
		An	Analysis
CN	**Client Need**		
Sa	Safe Effective Care Environment	**SA**	**Subject Area**
		1	Medical-Surgical
Sa/1	Management of Care	2	Psychiatric and Mental Health
Sa/2	Safety and Infection Control		
He/3	Health Promotion and Maintenance	3	Maternity and Women's Health
Ps/4	Psychosocial Integrity	4	Pediatric
Ph	Physiological Integrity	5	Pharmacologic
Ph/5	Basic Care and Comfort	6	Gerontologic
Ph/6	Pharmacological and Parenteral Therapies	7	Community Health
		8	Legal and Ethical Issues

Practice Test 1

1. In evaluating a client's success in learning relaxation techniques, the nurse will look for which the following behaviors?

    1. Experiencing anxiety without feeling overwhelmed
    2. Keeping a detailed journal of anxiety-provoking situations
    3. Reporting any anxious feelings to the nurse
    4. Regularly practicing progressive muscle relaxation

2. Which of the following short-term goals will the nurse select as priority for the client experiencing severe anxiety?

    1. Discover the precipitant of the anxiety
    2. Reduce the anxiety level
    3. Teach more effective coping skills
    4. Conduct a thorough assessment

3. While being evaluated for clinical manifestations consistent with panic attack, a client is concerned about the kind and number of laboratory tests ordered. The nurse most appropriately addresses the client's concern by explaining that

    1. panic attacks can only be definitively diagnosed through laboratory tests.
    2. laboratory tests can confirm the existence of panic attack.
    3. laboratory tests will identify the cause of panic attack.
    4. laboratory tests can discover conditions sharing the clinical manifestations of panic attack.

4. Which of the following questions would best help the nurse elicit the clinical manifestations of a social anxiety disorder?

   1. "Do you ever find yourself becoming anxious unexpectedly?"
   2. "Do you often check things repeatedly?"
   3. "Do you dread meeting new people?"
   4. "Do you tend to worry about many different things?"

5. In planning treatment activities, the nurse takes into account that the client with agoraphobia most fears

   1. being somewhere from which escape is difficult.
   2. meeting important people.
   3. having to repeat actions several times.
   4. small, furry animals.

6. In discussing the treatment plan with a client who has a specific phobia, the nurse properly emphasizes which of the following?

   1. In order to be successfully treated, the client must explore the precipitant for this fear
   2. It is vital that the client be involved in structuring the desensitization hierarchy
   3. Proficiency in self-hypnosis is essential to success in desensitization
   4. Specific phobia is more difficult to overcome than other anxiety disorders

7. During a day treatment program, a client newly diagnosed with social phobia attempts to avoid eating lunch with the rest of the group. The nurse can best help this client by

   1. insisting the client eat lunch with the group.
   2. offering the client a reward to eat lunch with the group.
   3. allowing the client to eat lunch in a private area.
   4. asking the client to write down feelings about eating with the group.

8. In discussing the use of monoamine oxidase inhibitors (MAOIs) with a client, the nurse emphasizes that the biggest complication with this class of drugs is _____.

9. A client newly diagnosed with panic disorder confides in the nurse, "I think I must be getting worse. I used to only have attacks in stores. Now I'm getting them in the cafeteria at work. I've started eating lunch at my desk because I'm afraid of having another attack." Which of the following would be the best initial response by the nurse?

1. "This is typically the way panic disorder progresses before treatment begins to be effective."

2. "The best thing you can do right now is to keep a detailed journal of when and where these attacks happen."

3. "Do you think it might be possible for you to take some time off from work?"

4. "I'm going to be teaching you some relaxation techniques to help with that."

10. One of the treatment goals for a client with generalized anxiety disorder is to recognize the onset of severe anxiety. The nurse knows the goal has been reached when the client states which of the following?

    1. "I've been feeling very little anxiety when I'm in group."

    2. "These relaxation exercises have helped such a lot."

    3. "I know what's happening now when my heart is racing."

    4. "I know now when to expect problems with anxiety."

11. The registered nurse on an inpatient unit is making out the day's assignment. There is a licensed practical nurse (LPN) on the team to whom some tasks may be delegated. Which of the following tasks are properly delegated to an LPN?

    1. Assessing the need for a p.r.n. anxiety medication

    2. Developing goals for a client's treatment plan

    3. Teaching a client progressive muscle relaxation

    4. Reviewing the dietary restrictions for a client on a monoamine oxidase inhibitor (MAOI)

12. The nurse is reviewing the treatment plan for a client with agoraphobia who has experienced some periods of panic-level anxiety. Which of the following nursing diagnoses would the nurse determine to be the priority?

    1. Coping, ineffective

    2. Role performance, ineffective

    3. Violence, risk for self-directed

    4. Social isolation

13. while making rounds, the nurse discovers that a client with a checking obsession has recently begun collecting empty milk cartons and other used containers from the meal trays. Which of the following are the most appropriate actions for the nurse to perform?Select all that apply:

    [ ] 1. Document the client's behavior as indicating increased anxiety

    [ ] 2. Review the client's treatment plan for possible revisions

    [ ] 3. Explain to the client that behavior at meals must now be monitored

[ ] **4.** Have the client wash out the cartons and containers

[ ] **5.** Have the client eat out of sight of the other clients

[ ] **6.** Tell the client to avoid collecting the milk containers

14. The nurse is explaining how cognitive reframing works to prepare a client with agoraphobia for a cognitive-behavioral therapy group when the client exclaims, "You're just like my family. You think this is all in my head." The best response on the nurse's part would be which of the following?

   1. "I think you're trying to tell me you're not ready for group."

   2. "Families never do seem to understand us, do they?"

   3. "I'm sorry. Let's continue this when you're feeling calmer."

   4. "Can we talk more about what you and your family know about agoraphobia?"

15. During visiting hours, one client's apparently blind visitor was accompanied to the unit by a service dog. Another client dashed shrieking from the visiting area and was found cowering in the restroom by the nurse. The priority action by the nurse at this time is to

   1. politely ask the person with the dog to leave.

   2. find a place perceived to be safe for the frightened client.

   3. explain the situation to the people in the visiting area.

   4. inform the frightened client's physician of this behavior.

16. An inpatient behavioral health unit employs some unlicensed assistive personnel. Which of the following activities may the nurse appropriately delegate to unlicensed assistive personnel?Select all that apply:

   [ ] **1.** Document the response of a client with social phobia to a cinema field trip

   [ ] **2.** Evaluate the effect of a client's relaxation practice on the level of anxiety reported

   [ ] **3.** Monitor a client's blood pressure after a new drug is given

   [ ] **4.** Plan the weekly current events for a client discussion group

   [ ] **5.** Teach the client about dietary restrictions

   [ ] **6.** Inform the client of the visiting hours

17. The parent of a child hit by a car arrives at the emergency room with streaming tears, visibly shaking, lamenting "Oh, my God, my baby!" loudly and repetitively, and trying to push by staff to see the child even though specifically asked to wait until x-rays are completed. The nurse assesses this parent's anxiety level as _____.

18. A general practice client expresses concern to the nurse about the physician having prescribed a beta blocker for tachycardia and palpitations when giving presentations at work. The client states, "My mother took that for her heart. Does the doctor think my anxiety might give me a heart attack?" Which of the following would be the nurse's best response to the client?

   1. "Oh, I'm sure that's not what the doctor thinks. I've seen this drug prescribed a lot for clients here."

   2. "The best person to ask about drugs is the pharmacist. That's who I always ask when I have questions."

   3. "I've seen your ECG and your heart looks fine. Did your mother have anxiety too?"

   4. "The purpose of beta blockers is to keep your heart from racing and pounding when you get nervous."

19. The nurse is talking to a student nurse who tells the nurse of feelings of anxiousness when taking examinations in school. The nurse informs the student nurse that this is what stage of anxiety? _____

20. The nurse assesses a client with a general anxiety disorder to have which of the following clinical manifestations?Select all that apply:

   [ ] 1. Irritability

   [ ] 2. Restlessness

   [ ] 3. Difficulty concentrating

   [ ] 4. Ritualistic behaviors

   [ ] 5. Hallucinatory-like flashbacks

   [ ] 6. Muscle tension

21. A client suspected of having a panic disorder tells the nurse of experiencing intense palpitations, sweating, shortness of breath, and chest pain when approaching the boarding gate to the airplane. The nurse evaluates which of the following characteristics as a priority in supporting this diagnosis?

   1. The client is able to verbalize personal feelings about flying

   2. The intense anxiety that peaks within 10 minutes of the stimuli

   3. A feeling of wanting to avoid flying altogether

   4. The client senses a feeling of impending doom

22. The nurse assesses which of the following clients to be at risk for developing a social phobia?

   1. A student who becomes anxious at the thought of taking an exam

   2. A client who suffered a stroke

   3. A hospitalized client

   4. A client who is afraid to leave home

23. Which of the following is a priority to consider before planning the care for a client who has obsessive-compulsive disorder?

    1. The client recognizes the behavior as unreasonable

    2. The client wishes to stop the behavior

    3. The client's ritualistic behavior should not be taken away until a substitute has been found to relieve the anxiety

    4. The client's behavior is motivated by a secondary gain for attention

24. The nurse is admitting a client who verbalizes feeling anxious after witnessing a car accident. The nurse should document this client as having what level of anxiety? _____

25. A client has been undergoing desensitization for a driving phobia. The nurse will know treatment has been successful when the client reports

    1. recognizing that the fear of driving is excessive and unrealistic.

    2. riding in the car with a friend.

    3. driving to the mall.

    4. planning a driving trip at AAA.

ANSWERS AND RATIONALES

1. **1.** Relaxation techniques reduce individuals' experience of anxiety to a tolerable level. Having the client keep a journal on anxiety-provoking situations and reporting anxious feelings to the nurse may perhaps be useful, but they do not specifically relate to the effective use of relaxation techniques. Although relaxation techniques are best mastered when regularly practiced, regular practice does not evaluate their effective use.
   NP = As
   CN = Ps/4
   CL = An
   SA = 2

2. **2.** Anxiety reduction is always the most important goal for all levels of anxiety above mild. Discovering the precipitant of anxiety, teaching more coping skills, and conducting a thorough assessment would not be appropriate because a severe level of anxiety prevents individuals from being able to effectively participate in any of these activities.
   NP = Pl
   CN = Ps/4
   CL = Ap
   SA = 2

3. 4. There are a number of conditions that share the same clinical manifestations as a panic attack. There are no laboratory tests that can diagnose, confirm, or discover the cause of panic attack.
NP = Ev
CN = Ps/4
CL = An
SA = 2

4. 3. Individuals with social phobia are most likely to avoid situations where they must interact with people. It would not be appropriate to ask a client with a social anxiety disorder if anxiety comes on unexpectedly because that question would be just as appropriate for a client with a panic disorder. Checking things repeatedly is an indication of obsessive-compulsive disorder. Worrying about many different things is a sign of a generalized anxiety disorder.
NP = An
CN = Ps/4
CL = An
SA = 2

5. 1. People with agoraphobia avoid venturing away from familiar, safe places. Being afraid of meeting people is a sign of a social phobia. A client who fears repeating things several times is displaying obsessive-compulsive disorder. A client who is afraid of small furry animals has a specific phobia.
NP = Pl
CN = Ps/4
CL = Ap
SA = 2

6. 2. Only clients can effectively rank the degree to which specific situations provoke anxiety for them. Identification of precipitants is seldom helpful in treatment. Relaxation ability in general, not self-hypnosis as a particular method of relaxation, is essential. Specific phobias respond more easily to treatment than some other anxiety disorders.
NP = Pl
CN = Ps/4
CL = An
SA = 2

7. 3. Allowing the client with a social phobia to eat in private will decrease anxiety and increase trust in staff. Confronting the client with an anxiety-provoking situation without a specific treatment plan is both cruel and counterproductive. Rewards will not help make the client more comfortable in the situation. Although it may be appropriate to write down feelings about eating with the group, it does not resolve the present situation.

NP = Im
CN = Ps/4
CL = Ap
SA = 2

8. **hypertensive crisis.** MAOIs inhibit the breakdown of tyramine in the body. If foods high in tyramine or sympathetomimetic drugs are concurrently consumed, the potential result is a dangerously high blood pressure response.
NP = Im
CN = Ps/4
CL = An
SA = 2

9. 1. The most helpful, anxiety-reducing first intervention is to educate the client about the course of the panic disorder. Although keeping a detailed journal may be included in treatment planning, it is not the most helpful response initially. Telling the client to take some time off from work reinforces the client's concern about "getting worse" and encourages more avoidance behavior. Although relaxation training may be included in treatment planning, it does not respond to the client's immediate concern.
NP = An
CN = Ps/4
CL = An
SA = 2

10. 3. Tachycardia is a physiological manifestation consistent with severe anxiety.
NP = Ev
CN = Ps/4
CL = An
SA = 2

11. 4. An LPN may review material that has already been taught to a client. It is inappropriate for a registered nurse (RN) to delegate tasks that involve assessment, planning, or initial teaching to an LPN.
NP = Pl
CN = Sa/1
CL = Ap
SA = 8

12. 3. Safety concerns are always the priority with agoraphobia, so risk for self-directed violence is the most appropriate diagnosis. Ineffective coping, ineffective role performance, and social isolation are important goals but must be deferred until client safety is addressed.

NP = Ev
CN = Ps/4
CL = An
SA = 2

13. 1, 2, 4. Hoarding is a variant of obsessive-compulsive behavior and its recent onset is an indication of escalating anxiety. Given a new clinical manifestation that indicates increased anxiety, the treatment plan will likely need modification. To remove the objects would only increase the client's anxiety further, but washing them will avoid problems with bugs and mold. There would be no benefit in monitoring mealtime behavior, because this may further increase the client's anxiety.
NP = Im
CN = Ps/4
CL = Ap
SA = 2

14. 4. A client who does not understand an illness cannot understand how any particular treatment might help with it. Deciding the client is not ready for group is a premature evaluation. Agreeing with the client that families do not understand is demeaning to the family, undermines their support, and doesn't address the client's concern. Postponing discussion with the client simply puts the client off and discourages further voicing of concerns.
NP = An
CN = Ps/4
CL = An
SA = 2

15. 2. Given the client's apparent level of fear at being in the presence of the dog, the priority is assuring the safety of that client. It is generally impermissible to bar service dogs from public places. Although explaining the situation to the visitors and informing the frightened client's physician are important actions, they can be completed after the safety of the frightened client is addressed.
NP = Im
CN = Ps/4
CL = Ap
SA = 2

16. 1, 3, 6. Unlicensed assistive personnel are trained to document behavior accurately. Monitoring vital signs and informing the client about visiting hours are within the capabilities and job description of unlicensed assistive personnel. Only a registered nurse (RN) can evaluate the effect of a treatment, such as relaxation techniques. The RN is the only one who can be responsible for planning therapeutic activities or teaching clients.

NP = Pl
CN = Sa/1
CL = Ap
SA = 8

17. **panic.** It is at panic level of anxiety that individuals lose behavioral control and have difficulty following verbal instruction.
NP = As
CN = Ps/4
CL = An
SA = 2

18. **4.** The most appropriate response for the nurse to give a client who thinks a beta blocker has been prescribed to prevent a heart attack is to explain the purpose of the beta blocker. This will alleviate the client's concerns. Telling a client that a lot of clients take beta blockers, to ask the pharmacist, or that the ECG looks fine all are interventions that put off the client's primary concern and are not appropriate.
NP = An
CN = Ps/4
CL = An
SA = 2

19. **Moderate.** Moderate anxiety focuses on the present concerns of the client. The perceptual field is narrowed and the client exhibits selective inattention.
NP = Im
CN = Ps/4
CL = An
SA = 2

20. **1, 2, 3, 6.** Clinical manifestations of a general anxiety disorder include irritability, restlessness, difficulty concentrating, fatigue, sleep disturbances, and muscle tension. Ritualistic behaviors occur in obsessive-compulsive disorders. Hallucinatory-like flashbacks are characteristic of post-traumatic disorders.
NP = As
CN = Ps/4
CL = An
SA = 2

21. **2.** Although it is a positive sign that a client with a panic disorder is able to verbalize personal feelings, the priority characteristic to support a diagnosis of a panic disorder is an intense anxiety within 10 minutes of the stimuli. The client may also want to avoid flying or may feel a sense of impending doom.

NP = Ev
CN = Ps/4
CL = An
SA = 2

22. 3. A hospitalized client may develop a social anxiety disorder. Clients who are in strange places with strange people may be afraid to speak up and address their concerns. A client who expresses anxiety prior to taking an exam is exhibiting a moderate anxiety. A client who suffered a stroke may be at risk for a general anxiety disorder. A client who is afraid to leave the home is experiencing agoraphobia.
NP = As
CN = Ps/4
CL = An
SA = 2

23. 3. Although a client with obsessive-compulsive disorder may want to stop the behavior and may recognize the behavior as unreasonable, it is a priority to consider not taking away the client's compulsive acts until the client has some other method to channel anxiety. A client with obsessive-compulsive disorder does not display the ritualistic behavior for a secondary gain.
NP = An
CN = Ps/4
CL = An
SA = 2

24. Severe. A client who has a severe anxiety level focuses on a specific detail, such as a car accident.
NP = As
CN = Ps/4
CL = An
SA = 2

25. 3. Desensitization is successful when the most fearful situation in the hierarchy of fears related to driving is encountered without undue anxiety. Although riding in the car with a friend and planning a trip are likely steps on a desensitization hierarchy, they are not the final goal. Phobic people typically recognize the excessiveness of their anxiety around the phobic stimulus.
NP = An
CN = Ps/4
CL = An
SA = 2

SOMATOFORM DISORDERS - COMPREHENSIVE EXAM

1. When assessing a client suspected of a somatoform disorder who complains of pain, it would be essential for the nurse to consider which of the following?

   1. The absence of laboratory findings to support the physical clinical manifestations

   2. The duration and intensity of the pain

   3. The performance of the client on reality testing

   4. The ability of the client to describe the precipitating factors

2. When planning care for a client with somatoform disorder, it is important for the nurse to include

   1. the option for alternative medicines.

   2. stress management strategies for the client.

   3. an antipsychotic drug.

   4. a behavior modification plan for the client's family.

3. The client's family asks the nurse what the chances are that the client will be able to recover from the somatoform disorder. The nurse's response should be based on an understanding of which of the following criteria?

   1. The etiology of the stress is the key to the cure

   2. The ability of the family to control the client's environment

   3. The client's psychological makeup

   4. The ability to establish a physical cause of the disorder

4. When interviewing a client with a somatoform disorder, it is a priority that the nurse understands which of the following characteristics about the disorder?

   1. The client is not aware that the etiology is psychological

   2. The client does not feel pain

   3. Manipulation of the nurse is the goal

   4. The client is helpless to control the environment

5. The client with somatization disorder presents with a unique set of clinical manifestations. The nurse makes which of the following assessments when collecting a nursing history from the client? The pain

   1. will come and go.

   2. is intense and localized.

   3. is felt in multiple sites.

   4. does not really exist.

6. The nurse is admitting a client who, on the day of a scheduled job interview, experienced a seizure. The electroencephalogram and medical workup are all negative. The client seems indifferent to the condition. The nurse reports this client as having what disorder? _____

7. A client comes into the emergency room complaining of pain. The nurse taking a history notices that the client has had numerous visits to the hospital, but no physical etiology for the pain has been found. This visit also does not validate a physical problem. The nurse should consider which of the following recommendations?

1. Psychiatric consultation for the possibility of a pain disorder

2. Administration of analgesics to help relieve the pain

3. A referral to physical therapy

4. A diagnosis of malingering in the client

8. When caring for a client with conversion disorder, one of the classic clinical manifestations that the nurse assesses is

1. a lack of concern about the disorder.

2. an extreme anxiousness about the disorder.

3. an unawareness of the disorder.

4. a chronic disorder that escalates in severity.

9. Which of the following assessments would provide the nurse with the most accurate information regarding the client's pain disorder?

1. Preoccupation with an imagined defect in appearance

2. Occurrence of pain in one or more anatomical sites

3. Presence of one or more clinical manifestations suggesting neurological or medical disorder

4. Pain not associated with psychological or medical disorder

10. Which of the following factors must the nurse rule out when collecting a nursing history on a 20-year-old client with a somatoform disorder?

1. The disorder had an onset before 30 years of age

2. Unresolved guilt is the etiology

3. The existence of a single physical complaint

4. Multiple complaints unsubstantiated by lab tests

11. A client diagnosed with hypochondriasis is admitted to the psychiatric unit. The nurse planning the care should include which of the following in the plan of care?

1. Develop a relationship that allows for identification of anxiety-producing events

2. Inform the client that the clinical manifestations are imagined

3. Administer the drug to control the discomfort of the disorder

4. Use behavior modification techniques to extinguish the abnormal behavior

12. When treating a client with a pain disorder, the nurse should include which of the following treatment measures as a priority?

1. Administer drugs for pain to alleviate the discomfort

2. Help the client identify somatic clinical manifestations as coping strategies

3. Avoid the client's complaints of pain

4. Identify the family dynamics that make the client sick

13. The nurse working with a client who has a body dysmorphic disorder complains of being extremely fat. The nurse would know that it is important to implement which of the following measures into the client's care plan?

1. A referral to a plastic surgeon

2. Opportunity for social interaction

3. Strict low-caloric diet

4. Rigorous exercise regime

14. A client is admitted to the psychiatric unit, having developed a sudden limping gait. Which of the following diagnostic criteria must be present before the diagnosis of a conversion disorder can be made?

1. The client suffered a traumatic injury that precipitated the impairment

2. The clinical manifestations are feigned for attention

3. The client is indifferent to the condition

4. The client is extremely preoccupied with the condition

15. The nurse is working with a client diagnosed with factitious disorder. In order to plan for appropriate care, which of the following criteria is imperative to understand?

1. The client does not perceive the disorder as real

2. The client receives secondary gain from the disorder

3. The clinical manifestations are outside of the client's control

4. Drug therapy is essential to control the clinical manifestations

16. What behavior characteristics does the client exhibit when a diagnosis of malingering is made? _____

17. The nurse informs another nurse that which of the following feelings may be present in the nurse caring for a client with a conversion disorder?

1. Empathy

2. Sympathy

3. Anger

4. Sadness

18. The nurse is caring for a client with a somatoform disorder. To optimize the treatment goal, which of the following should be included in the client's plan of care?

    1. Avoid focusing on the stressors

    2. Encourage the client to identify somatic clinical manifestations

    3. Encourage the family to adapt to the client's behavior

    4. Implement a drug regime for the client

19. The nurse evaluates a client with a conversion disorder to have which of the following characteristics?Select all that apply:

    [ ] 1. Clinical manifestations are intentionally produced

    [ ] 2. Clinical manifestations suggest a neurological or medical condition

    [ ] 3. Deficit does not cause significant distress

    [ ] 4. Deficit is not limited to pain or sexual dysfunction

    [ ] 5. Clinical manifestations are not fully explained by a medical condition

    [ ] 6. Deficit occurs independent of a somatization disorder

20. The nurse identifies which of the following as the primary feature that separates factitious disorders from other somatoform disorders?

    1. Clinical manifestations are intentional

    2. Physical or psychological clinical manifestations occur to gain attention

    3. At least four pain clinical manifestations must be present

    4. Physical or psychological clinical manifestations cannot be explained by medical condition

21. Which of the following observations would best indicate that the treatment plan for a client with a body dysmorphic disorder has been successful?

    1. The client is becoming less withdrawn and less isolated

    2. The client is taking care of grooming needs

    3. The client is less preoccupied with appearance

    4. The client no longer is seeking surgical intervention

22. When developing a treatment plan for a client with Munchausen syndrome, the nurse includes which of the following measures?

    1. Pay close attention to the progress of the reported illness

    2. Avoid focusing on the clinical manifestations

3. Instruct the client on the appropriate measures for meeting emotional needs

4. Administer drugs to control the clinical manifestations of distress

23. When evaluating the progress of the client with a pain disorder, which of the following would indicate to the nurse that the client is improving? The client

   1. understands the link between the pain and the conflict.

   2. learns to control the clinical manifestations with drug therapy.

   3. avoids focusing on the pain.

   4. has a decrease in the number of health care visits.

24. When treating a client with a pain disorder, it is essential that the nurse encourage which of the following measures?

   1. Routine health care visits

   2. Drug therapy

   3. Social interaction

   4. Referral for pain management

25. The nurse is caring for a female client who is convinced she has a serious condition that has gone undiagnosed. Which of the following must be present for successful treatment? Select all that apply:

   [ ] 1. Trust in the health care providers

   [ ] 2. Decreased depression

   [ ] 3. Reassurance regarding physical health

   [ ] 4. Understanding of how the perception of the body leads to an overemphasis of illness

   [ ] 5. Use of antidepressants

   [ ] 6. Hypnotherapy

26. The registered nurse is preparing the clinical assignments on a psychiatric unit. Which of the following assignments should the nurse delegate to a licensed practical nurse?

   1. Teach a class on somatoform disorders to new personnel on the unit

   2. Instruct a client with a body dysmorphic disorder on eating a well-balanced diet

   3. Administer a selective serotonin reuptake inhibitor to a client with hypochondriasis

   4. Assess a client with a somatization disorder for clinical manifestations

ANSWERS AND RATIONALES

1. 1. One of the key criteria for the diagnosis of somatoform disorder is the absence of laboratory findings to support physical clinical manifestations. Duration and intensity of pain could be from physical clinical manifestations. Reality testing is not a factor because clients with the disorder are nondelusional. The etiology of the disorder is psychological and out of the awareness of the client.
NP = An
CN = Ps/4
CL = An
SA = 2

2. 2. Stress precipitates and exacerbates somatoform disorder. Alternative medicines are not proven to help in somatoform disorder. The disorder does not produce psychotic episodes; therefore, antipsychotics are inappropriate. Behavior modification would be used by the client, not the client's family.
NP = Pl
CN = Ps/4
CL = Ap
SA = 2

3. 3. One of the best indicators for prediction of recovery is the client's psychological makeup and the ability to deal with the underlying emotional components. Stress is a precipitant of pain, but if the client cannot deal with the stress there will not be recovery from the disorder. The etiology of the pain is psychological.
NP = An
CN = Ps/4
CL = An
SA = 2

4. 1. The criterion of somatoform disorder is that it is of psychological etiology. The client does feel pain. Manipulation is not the goal in a true somatoform disorder as it is in factitious disorder or malingering. The client does have control of the environment.
NP = An
CN = Ps/4
CL = An
SA = 2

5. 3. The pain in a somatization disorder is felt in four or more sites. The pain may be constant, not localized, and it really exists.
NP = As
CN = Ps/4

CL = An
SA = 2

6. **Conversion disorder.** In a conversion disorder, there are one or more clinical manifestations suggesting a neurological or medical disorder. The clinical manifestations are associated with a psychological stressor, such as a job interview. An indifference to the condition is generally exhibited.
NP = An
CN = Ps/4
CL = An
SA = 2

7. 1. The nurse who encounters a client with multiple hospital visits and no established diagnosis should consider the possibility of a pain disorder. Because dependence on analgesics is to be avoided, drugs are used only if there is sufficient diagnostic evidence. Referral to physical therapy is also contingent upon a physical disorder. Malingering should be diagnosed only after a pain disorder is ruled out.
NP = Ev
CN = Ps/4
CL = An
SA = 2

8. 1. The classic feature of a conversion disorder is that the client does not feel distressed with it. The client is unconcerned and not anxious. The disorder is within the client's awareness. The disorder is short term and remits when the conflict resolves.
NP = As
CN = Ps/4
CL = An
SA = 2

9. 2. There is pain in one or more anatomical sites with a pain disorder. The pain may be associated with a psychological or medical disorder. Preoccupation with an imagined defect in appearance is a body dysmorphic disorder. Clinical manifestations suggesting a neurological or medical disorder is called a conversion disorder.
NP = As
CN = Ps/4
CL = An
SA = 2

10. 3. Somatoform disorder has four or more sites of pain. The existence of one physical complaint is not consistent with a diagnosis of a somatoform disorder. Onset of the disorder is before 30 years of age and therefore supports the diagnosis and cannot be ruled out. Unresolved guilt is the

etiology. Multiple complaints unsubstantiated by lab tests is another criterion for establishing the diagnosis.

NP = Ev
CN = Ps/4
CL = An
SA = 2

11. 1. A key component for care of the client with hypochondriasis is the development of a therapeutic alliance or relationship. Informing the client that clinical manifestations are a result of the imagination will only exacerbate the manifestations. Drugs should be administered judiciously, because the etiology of the problem is not physical. The use of behavior modification will not extinguish the behavior, because the etiology is psychological.

NP = Pl
CN = Ps/4
CL = Ap
SA = 2

12. 2. The identification of somatic clinical manifestations and coping strategies are pivotal for recovery. Drugs for pain can lead to dependence. The client's concerns need to be addressed to help to resolve the disorder. Family issues are dealt with later in the therapeutic process.

NP = Pl
CN = Sa/1
CL = Ap
SA = 2

13. 2. Opportunity for social interaction is crucial because the client with a body dysmorphic disorder tends to withdraw and become isolated. A referral to a plastic surgeon supports the client's misinterpretation about appearance. Extreme dieting is one of the dangers for the client who feels overweight when within normal weight range. Rigorous exercise is also a danger if clients feel that they are overweight, because it reinforces a false body image.

NP = Im
CN = Ps/4
CL = Ap
SA = 2

14. 3. The client's indifference is a classic manifestation of a conversion disorder. The client who had a traumatic injury would have a physical etiology for the clinical manifestations. The clinical manifestations are not to gain attention. The client is not concerned about the appearance of the clinical manifestations.

NP = Ev
CN = Ps/4
CL = An
SA = 2

15. 2. The client with factitious disorder has a primary need for secondary gain that reinforces the disorder. The client's disorder may be real or feigned. The clinical manifestations are within the client's control. Drug therapy is not appropriate for control of the clinical manifestations.
NP = An
CN = Ps/4
CL = An
SA = 2

16. Attention-seeking behaviors. Attention-seeking behavior is a key diagnostic criterion for malingering.
NP = Ev
CN = Ps/4
CL = An
SA = 2

17. 3. It is not unusual for the nurse to foster feelings of anger when caring for a client with a conversion disorder. The nurse must learn to deal with the client objectively and without confrontation.
NP = Im
CN =Ps/4
CL = An
SA = 2

18. 2. The ability to identify somatic clinical manifestations is the first step in recovery from a somatoform disorder. The client who tries to ignore the stressors will only exacerbate them. The family needs to help the client change the behaviors as well as the stressors. Drug therapy is generally not used because it creates dependence.
NP = Ev
CN = Ps/4
CL = An
SA = 2

19. 2, 4, 5. A conversion disorder involves one or more clinical manifestations, suggesting a neurological or medical condition. The clinical manifestations are not intentionally produced or explained by a medical condition. The deficit causes significant distress, is not limited to pain or sexual dysfunction, and does not occur independent of the somatoform disorder.
NP = Ev
CN = Ps/4

CL = An
SA = 2

20. 1. With a factitious disorder, there is an intentional effort on the part of the client to produce physical or psychological manifestations to gain attention. As with all other somatoform disorders, at least four pain clinical manifestations must be present, and the clinical manifestations are not explained by a medical condition.
NP = An
CN = Sa/1
CL = An
SA = 2

21. 3. A client who has a body dysmorphic disorder will have made progress when there is a decrease in the preoccupation with appearance. Although a client who is less withdrawn and isolated is making progress, the best indication of successful treatment with a body dysmorphic disorder is the reduced preoccupation with appearance.
NP = Ev
CN = Ps/4
CL = An
SA = 2

22. 3. Implementing the appropriate measures for meeting the emotional needs of a client with Munchausen syndrome will allow the client to control the clinical manifestations. Attention to the feigned clinical manifestations results in secondary gain. Ignoring the clinical manifestations will escalate the behavior. Drug therapy is not indicated for Munchausen syndrome.
NP = Pl
CN = Ps/4
CL = Ap
SA = 2

23. 1. The ability of the client to link pain with conflict is the key to cure a pain disorder. Drugs for pain put the client at risk for dependence. The client should not ignore the pain but try to deal with the psychological etiology. Routine and regularly scheduled health care visits are a sign of progress.
NP = Ev
CN = Ps/4
CL = An
SA = 2

24. 1. Routine health care visits allow the client with a pain disorder to become confident that physical health is being monitored. Drugs for pain are to be avoided because of dependence. Social interaction is not usually a

problem for the client with a pain disorder; such a client is seeking attention with the pain clinical manifestations. Since pain is not of a physical etiology, it is inappropriate to use medical measures to manage the disorder.

NP = Pl
CN = Ps/4
CL = Ap
SA = 2

25. 1, 3, 4. Imperative to successful treatment in a somatoform disorder are a trust in health care providers, reassurance regarding a healthy physical state, and an understanding of how one's own perception of the body leads to an overwhelming sense of physical illness. Depression is not a classic feature. Antianxiety drugs, not antidepressants, may be used in the treatment because somatoform disorders share several characteristics with anxiety disorders. Hypnotherapy is used for dissociative disorders.

NP = Ev
CN = Ps/4
CL = An
SA = 2

26. 3. Teaching a class, instructing a client, and assessing a client are all tasks that require the skills of a registered nurse. A licensed practical nurse may administer oral drugs.

NP = Pl
CN = Sa/1
CL = An
SA = 8

DISSOCIATIVE DISORDERS - COMPREHENSIVE EXAM

1. The nurse evaluates which of the following statements to best describe dissociative disorders? Dissociative disorders

   1. are fixed and chronic.

   2. appear only in bipolar disorder.

   3. are feigned.

   4. are a result of anxiety.

2. A client is admitted to the psychiatric unit of the hospital with complaints of waking up in a strange location. The nurse who is assessing the client history concludes that this client suffers from what disorder?
_____

3. The nurse is taking the history from a client with dissociative amnesia. Which of the following findings in the history is significant?

   1. The client has a brain tumor

   2. The client actively abuses substances

   3. The client experiences forgetfulness

   4. The client is unable to recall personal information surrounding a traumatic event

4. A client's family asks the nurse what the purpose of the hypnotherapy is for a dissociative disorder. Which of the following is the most appropriate response by the nurse? "Hypnotherapy

   1. assists the client to reduce role strain."

   2. promotes a safe environment."

   3. develops triggers necessary to interrupt the dissociation episode."

   4. facilitates the retrieval of material from the consciousness."

5. When planning the care for a client with dissociative identity disorder, which one of the following measures is critical?

   1. Reestablish the client's true identity

   2. Encourage the emergence of all the personalities

   3. Ensure that the client's safety needs are met

   4. Discuss the characteristics of the different personalities

6. The nurse is caring for a client with a dissociative disorder who is experiencing alterations in consciousness, memory, or identity. The nurse evaluates which of the following nursing diagnoses to be most appropriate for this client?

   1. Ineffective coping

   2. Anxiety

   3. Interrupted family processes

   4. Ineffective role performance

7. The nurse is caring for a client with a dissociative disorder. Which of the following goals is a priority?

   1. The establishment of a therapeutic alliance

   2. The administration of psychotropic medications

   3. Development of knowledge of the content of the repressed information

   4. The ability to use hypnosis to uncover repressed feelings

8. When working with a client with depersonalization disorder, the nurse would most likely observe which of the following clinical manifestations in the client? Select all that apply:

[   ] **1.** Intact reality testing

[   ] **2.** Feelings of sadness

[   ] **3.** Impaired social or occupational functioning

[   ] **4.** Substance abuse

[   ] **5.** Feelings of rage

[   ] **6.** Feelings of detachment

9. The nurse is admitting a client with a dissociative disorder who is extremely depressed and suicidal. Which of the following is a priority for the nurse to include in this client's plan of care?

   1. Hypnotherapy

   2. Family counseling

   3. Milieu therapy

   4. Psychotherapy

10. The nurse attempts to assist a client with a dissociative disorder to see the consequences of using dissociation to cope. The client becomes angry and asks the nurse why. The most appropriate response by the nurse is which of the following?

    1. "It is important that you see the absurdity of your behavior."

    2. "It increases your insight and helps you understand your behavior."

    3. "You need to know there is no benefit to your behavior."

    4. "It will decrease your anxiety."

11. The nurse is collecting a nursing history from a client admitted with dissociative identity disorder. Which of the following questions should the nurse ask?

    1. "Were you abused physically or sexually as a child?"

    2. "Did you have an early developmental delay?"

    3. "Have you ever experienced hallucinations?"

    4. "Do you frequently travel away from a common location?"

12. When interviewing a client, the client complains to the nurse of feeling not human. The nurse reports that this client is experiencing what disorder?

_____

13. The nurse identifies which of the following tasks to be frustrating for a client who has dissociative amnesia?

    1. Recalling the activities surrounding a traumatic event

    2. Carrying out activities of daily living

    3. Remembering personal information from the remote past

    4. Writing in a journal

14. The nurse planning for the care of the client with dissociative identity disorder would include which of the following measures?
    1. Forcing the client to remember the traumatic past
    2. Telling the client about the existence of subpersonalities
    3. Encouraging time alone to promote recall
    4. Simplifying the client's daily routines

15. Which of the following nursing diagnoses would be appropriate for a client with a dissociative disorder who is in an altered state and unable to explain behaviors?
    1. Anxiety
    2. Spiritual distress
    3. Disturbed personal identity
    4. Risk for self-directed violence

16. Which of the following is a priority before the diagnosis of a dissociative disorder can be made?
    1. Rule out any medical condition
    2. Ask the client if feelings of anxiousness are present
    3. Evaluate for the presence of depression
    4. Obtain a family history

17. Which of the following would be an indication that positive progress is being made when working with a client who has dissociative identity disorder?
    1. The disappearance of subpersonalities
    2. The control of rage episodes
    3. The ability to recognize hallucinations
    4. Positive responses to antipsychotics

18. The client with a long-term dissociative disorder may experience secondary clinical manifestations. What manifestations would be most important for the nurse to assess?
    1. Poor grooming
    2. Self-harm
    3. Failure of the memory to return
    4. Assumption of a new identity

19. The nurse is caring for a client who has an inability to recall information and is experiencing significant distress in both occupational and social life. The nurse documents that this client is experiencing what disorder?

20. A nurse is conducting an intake assessment on a client suspected of depersonalization disorder. Which of the following clinical manifestations is the diagnostic criterion for this disorder?

    1. Obsessional thinking of past events

    2. Sensations of being detached

    3. Inability to recognize family members

    4. Difficulties do not occur in the work environment

21. Which of the following is a priority question for the nurse to ask a client with dissociative identity disorder?

    1. "Do you enjoy meeting people?"

    2. "Are you afraid of heights?"

    3. "Do you ever find strange clothes in your closet?"

    4. "Do you enjoy your spare time?"

22. Which of the following interventions should the client include in the plan of care for a client with a dissociative disorder?Select all that apply:

    [ ] 1. Provide the client with a detailed routine

    [ ] 2. Avoid letting the client make personal decisions

    [ ] 3. Inform the client about past events

    [ ] 4. Allow the client to move at his or her own pace remembering events

    [ ] 5. Accept the client's expression of negative feelings

    [ ] 6. Instruct the client on stress-relieving techniques

23. Before planning the care for a client with dissociative fugue, the nurse should consider which of the following aspects?

    1. The disorder only abates with therapy

    2. The disorder may resolve by itself

    3. The disorder does not alter the client's memory

    4. The disorder is controlled by the client

24. The nurse working with a client with dissociative identity disorder should plan care that would take into account which of the following factors?

    1. The client was confronted with an intolerable terror event

    2. The dissociative episodes are known to the primary personality

    3. Control of the subpersonalities lies within the primary personality

    4. The client should be informed about all subpersonalities

25. A client's wife asks the nurse what is the other name for dissociative identity disorder. What is the appropriate response by the nurse?

26. The registered nurse is preparing to delegate clinical assignments on a psychiatric unit.Which of the following assignments should the nurse delegate to a licensed practical nurse?

   1. Develop a plan of care for a client admitted with dissociative fugue

   2. Obtain a nursing history from a client suspected of having dissociative amnesia

   3. Administer a psychotropic drug to a client with a dissociative disorder

   4. Create the nursing diagnoses for a client with dissociative identity disorder

ANSWERS AND RATIONALES

1. **4.** Dissociative disorders include a group of disorders that involve a disturbance in the organization of memory, identity, consciousness, and perception and are a result of anxiety. They are often short term and resolve on their own. They do not appear in bipolar disorders nor are they feigned.
   NP = Ev
   CN = Ps/4
   CL = An
   SA = 2

2. **Dissociative fugue.** Dissociative fugue is a dissociative disorder characterized by waking up in a strange location.
   NP = An
   CN = Ps/4
   CL = Co
   SA = 2

3. **4.** The inability to recall personal information surrounding a traumatic event would meet the diagnostic criterion for dissociative amnesia. The abuse of substances is a disqualifier for dissociative amnesia. A history of brain tumor is not significant in a client with dissociative amnesia. To meet the criterion for the disorder, the episodes cannot be attributable to common forgetfulness.
   NP = As
   CN = Ps/4
   CL = An
   SA = 2

4. **4.** Family counseling assists the client to reduce role strain. Milieu therapy promotes a safe environment. Identifying the triggers to dissociation and developing a plan to interrupt the dissociation process are coping skills that can be learned. Hypnotherapy frequently used in a dissociative

disorder encourages the client to relax so that the therapist can retrieve material from the unconsciousness.
NP = An
CN = Ps/4
CL = An
SA = 2

5. 3. Safety needs are always the primary concern for clients with dissociative identity disorder. The emergence of the personalities should not be encouraged by anyone other than the psychotherapist. The different personalities are for the therapist to discuss with the client; discussion of them lies outside the role of the generalist nurse.
NP = Pl
CN = Ps/4
CL = An
SA = 2

6. 1. Ineffective coping is the most appropriate nursing diagnosis for a client with a dissociative disorder. This client is experiencing alterations in consciousness, memory, or identity.
NP = Ev
CN = Ps/4
CL = An
SA = 2

7. 1. The establishment of a therapeutic alliance is a primary goal for the nurse working with a client who has a dissociative disorder. Administration of psychotropic medications may not be the appropriate pharmacologic agent. Knowledge of the content of the repressed information is not crucial for the nurse to know. Hypnosis is within the role of the therapist and is still unproven as a remedy.
NP = Pl
CN = Sa/1
CL = An
SA = 2

8. 1, 3, 6. Feelings of detachment, intact reality testing, and impaired social or occupational functioning are classic manifestations of depersonalization disorder. Feelings of sadness and rage are not seen in depersonalization disorder.
NP = As
CN = Ps/4
CL = Ap
SA = 2

9. 3. The priority for a client with a dissociative disorder who is depressed and suicidal is milieu therapy. A client who is suicidal may require

hospitalization. Safety is the priority. Hospitalization can provide a structured and supportive environment.

NP = Pl

CN = Sa/1

CL = An

SA = 2

10. **2.** The most appropriate response to a client who asks the nurse why the issue of dissociation is being discussed as a method of coping is that it increases insight and helps to develop an understanding of behavior. Indirectly, it may decrease the client's anxiety.

NP = An

CN = Ps/4

CL = An

SA = 2

11. **1.** A prior history of child abuse is one of the primary precipitating factors correlating with dissociative identity disorder. Early developmental delay may be a result of child abuse but is not the precipitating event. Hallucination is not a key component of dissociative identity disorder. Travel away from a common location is characteristic of dissociative fugue.

NP = As

CN = Ps/4

CL = An

SA = 2

12. **Dissociative identity disorder.** One of the classic manifestations of dissociative identity disorder is the feeling of not feeling human.

NP = An

CN = Ps/4

CL = Ap

SA = 2

13. **1.** Recalling is very difficult, if not impossible, because the memory of the client is blocked as a way to deal with the trauma. There is no difficulty with carrying out daily activities. Remembering remote personal information is not a problem. Only the events surrounding the trauma are blocked. Writing in a journal is a recommendation for the client with dissociative amnesia.

NP = An

CN = Ps/4

CL = An

SA = 2

14. **4.** The simpler the client's routines, the less frustrating and more therapeutic the client will find the environment. Forcing the client to remember only increases the clinical manifestations of dissociative

identity disorder. Informing the client of the existence of the subpersonalities is the responsibility of the psychotherapist and not the nurse. Isolation and withdrawal may cause problems and should be avoided.

NP = Pl

CN = Ps/4

CL = Ap

SA = 2

15. 4. The appropriate nursing diagnosis for a client with a dissociative disorder, in an altered state and unable to explain behaviors is Risk for self-directed violence.

NP = An

CN = Ps/4

CL = An

SA = 2

16. 1. Before the diagnosis of a dissociative disorder can be made, the presence of any physical or psychological condition must be ruled out. The client may feel anxious or be depressed as a result of the dissociative disorder. It may prove helpful to obtain a family history after the diagnosis of a dissociative disorder is made.

NP = Pl

CN = Sa/1

CL = An

SA = 2

17. 1. The disappearance of subpersonalities is a marker of progress in a client with dissociative identity disorder. Rage episodes and hallucinations are not characteristic. Antipsychotics are not recommended, because psychotic features are not part of the disorder.

NP = Ev

CN = Ps/4

CL = An

SA = 2

18. 2. The priority is self-harm. A client who has a dissociative disorder may experience the potential secondary problem of having a subpersonality try to rid the client of the primary personality. The client's grooming is important but does not supersede a suicide threat. The client's memory may or may not return. Clients often assume new identities.

NP = As

CN = Ps/4

CL = An

SA = 2

19. Dissociative amnesia. Dissociative amnesia is a dissociative disorder characterized by an inability to recall information often associated with a trauma or stress. It generally causes significant distress in both occupational and social life.
NP = An
CN = Ps/4
CL = Ap
SA = 2

20. 2. The sensation of being detached or nonhuman is an indication of depersonalization disorder. Obsession over past events is not a criterion. The inability to recognize family members is not generally a part of the disorder. Difficulties in the work environment occur as a result of the disorder.
NP = As
CN = Ps/4
CL = Ap
SA = 2

21. 3. A classic feature of dissociative identity disorder is finding clothes in the closet that are not recognized or talking to strangers as if they are old friends.
NP = As
CN = Sa/1
CL = Ap
SA = 2

22. 4, 5, ,6. Interventions to include in the plan of care for a client who has a dissociative disorder include allowing the client to choose a personal pace to remember events, accepting the client's expression of negative feelings, and instructing the client on stress-relieving techniques. The client should be provided with a simple routine that is nondemanding. The client should be encouraged to make the decisions if they are not too stress provoking. The client should also not be flooded with the events of the past.
NP = Pl
CN = Ps/4
CL = Ap
SA = 2

23. 2. Dissociative fugue often resolves by itself. The disorder does not always need therapy or drugs. The client often loses parts of the memory. The disorder is out of the control of the client.
NP = Pl
CN = Ps/4
CL = An
SA = 2

24. 1. The client represses traumatic events in dissociative identity disorder, and thus confrontation with such trauma is a precipitating factor. The dissociative episode is not known to the primary personality. The primary personality does not control the subpersonalities. The client needs to discover the existence of subpersonalities in therapy.
NP = Pl
CN = Ps/4
CL = An
SA = 2

25. **Multiple personality disorder.** Dissociative identity disorder used to be called multiple personality disorder.
NP = An
CN = Ps/4
CL = Co
SA = 2

26. 3. Developing a plan of care, obtaining a nursing history, and creating nursing diagnoses are all tasks that should be performed by a registered nurse. A licensed practical nurse may administer a drug.
NP = Pl
CN = Sa/1
CL = An

PERSONALITY DISORDERS - COMPREHENSIVE EXAM

1. The nurse is admitting a client who appears detached, has a flat affect, lacks close friends, shows emotional coldness, and expresses little interest in socialization and sex. The nurse documents this client as having what disorder? _____

2. Which of the following clinical manifestations would provide the nurse with the most accurate information regarding a client with paranoid personality disorder?Select all that apply:

   [ ] 1. Perception that others are attacking

   [ ] 2. Views self as special and unique

   [ ] 3. Suspicious of others

   [ ] 4. Preoccupied with power

   [ ] 5. Views relationships as closer than they are

   [ ] 6. Persistently bears grudges

3. When conducting a chart review, the nurse would find the clinical manifestations of borderline personality disorder in what age group? _____

4. A client who is being admitted tells the nurse about personal plans that include going into the military to be able to shoot guns and "blow people away." The nurse assesses this client to have blatant disregard of others, frequent episodes of lying, and failure to maintain permanent employment. The nurse should report this client to have what disorder? _____

ANSWERS AND RATIONALES

1. **Schizoid personality disorder.** Schizoid personality disorder is a personality disorder in which clients have a marked detachment from people and events. They spend a lot of time by themselves, lack close friends, show emotional coldness, and are indifferent to praise.
   NP = Im
   CN = Ps/4
   CL = Ap
   SA = 2

2. **1, 3, 6.** Essential features of paranoid personality disorders include an intense fear of others and their motives. Such a client perceives being attacked by other people and bears persistent grudges. A client who views oneself as special and unique and is preoccupied with power has narcissistic personality disorder. A client who views relationships as closer than they are has histrionic personality disorder.
   NP = As
   CN = Ps/4
   CL = Ap
   SA = 2

3. **Late adolescence to early adulthood.** Personality disorders including borderline personality disorder generally appear in late adolescence to early adulthood.
   NP = An
   CN = Ps/4
   CL = Ap
   SA = 2

4. **Antisocial personality disorder.** A client who has antisocial personality disorder has a pervasive pattern of disregard for and violation of the rights of others. The client generally has a predisposition to violence, blatant disregard for the safety of others, and is frequently in trouble with the law. The client tends to have trouble maintaining employment and repeatedly lies.
   NP = An
   CN = Ps/4
   CL = Ap
   SA = 2

Practice Test 2

1. A nurse is assigned to care for a client with a diagnosis of histrionic personality disorder. Which of the following clinical manifestations would the nurse anticipate finding?
Select all that apply:

[ ] 1. Lack of empathy toward others

[ ] 2. Impressionistic style of speech

[ ] 3. Reassurance seeking

[ ] 4. Wants to be the center of attention

[ ] 5. Has rapid shifts of emotions

[ ] 6. Exhibits rage and impulsive behavior

2. An emergency room nurse begins taking a history from a male client brought to the emergency room by the police after a fight with his girlfriend. The client speaks very highly of himself, behaves condescendingly to the nurse, and disregards the effect of his behavior and fight with his girlfriend. The nurse should plan the care for this client based on which of the following diagnoses?

1. Histrionic personality disorder

2. Borderline personality disorder

3. Avoidant personality disorder

4. Narcissistic personality disorder

3. The nurse is collecting a history on a client suspected of having antisocial personality disorder. Which of the following findings should the nurse report to support this diagnosis?
Select all that apply:

[   ] **1.** Lack of remorse

[   ] **2.** Disregard for the law

[   ] **3.** Requires admiration

[   ] **4.** Has an exaggerated range of emotions

[   ] **5.** Sense of impulsiveness

[   ] **6.** Uses physical appearance to draw attention to self

4. A nurse would find it difficult to engage a client with avoidant personality disorder based on which of the following?

1. Lack of empathy toward others

2. Lack of interest in pleasurable activities

3. Fear of being the target of others

4. Fear of embarrassment prevents trying new things

5. The nurse reviews an assignment for a client with a diagnosis of avoidant personality disorder. Which of the following should the nurse consider when planning care for the client?

1. The client agrees to let others assume responsibility

2. The client will be fearful of rejection

3. The client will not desire a close relationship with the nurse

4. The client will perceive the situation as a threat

6. Which of the following should the nurse include to engage a client with avoidant personality disorder?

1. Bring the client to a therapeutic group and encourage group members to challenge the client's irrational thoughts

2. Provide open opportunities for the client to seek out the nurse

3. Help the client

4. Support the client's reluctance to engage in self-determination

7. A client presents to the emergency department with complaints of stomach pain, fear of being alone, and seeking reassurance and nurturing from all staff. The nurse notifies the physician that this client has a probable diagnosis of _____.

8. The nurse caring for a client following a mastectomy notices the client is highly rigid with the placement of objects in the room and in considerable anxiety when that order is disturbed. The nurse should take what disorder into consideration before planning the care for this client? _____

9. A client's family member asks the nurse about the differences between paranoid schizophrenia and paranoid personality disorder. Which of the following is the appropriate response by the nurse?

1. "A client with paranoid personality disorder will exhibit behavior that is considered bizarre and irrational."

2. "With paranoid schizophrenia, the illness can often be traced to adolescence before remaining relatively stable."

3. "Hallucinations and delusions are common in both paranoid personality disorder and paranoid schizophrenia."

4. "Characteristics such as distrust and suspicion are common in both paranoid schizophrenia and paranoid personality disorder."

10. The nurse should include which of the following when planning care for a client with narcissistic personality disorder?

   1. Promote rapport by showing interest in the client's stories

   2. Limit interactions with the client

   3. Decrease the tendency for embellishment by acknowledging that the client is better than others

   4. Use reality focus, which occurs by challenging the client's misrepresentations

11. Which of the following should the nurse include when planning care for a client with avoidant personality disorder?

   1. Allow the client to stay in the room until the client feels comfortable with people

   2. Avoid acknowledging goals achieved by the client

   3. Enable the client to set and drive the goals independent of the nurse

   4. Promote self-esteem by praising the client's success

12. Which of the following clinical manifestations is a priority for the nurse to consider before planning the care of a client with a diagnosis of obsessive-compulsive personality disorder?

   1. Preoccupation with details

   2. Indecisiveness

   3. Reluctance to delegate tasks

   4. Envious of others

13. The nurse is caring for a client who complains of having trouble completing tasks on the job because the client wants the job done perfectly and fears getting fired. The nurse understands that the client is experiencing which of the following disorders?

   1. Dependent personality disorder

   2. Narcissistic personality disorder

   3. Obsessive-compulsive personality disorder

   4. Paranoid personality disorder

14. Which of the following characteristics should the nurse consider before planning ongoing measures associated with dependent personality disorder?

    1. They are eager to become involved in a therapeutic relationship because there is a sense of attachment

    2. They are eager to tell their story and have others admire what they have accomplished in the past

    3. They view a therapeutic relationship as a waste of time because they don't see a problem with their behavior

    4. They may vacillate between wanting the therapeutic relationship and pushing it away, dependent on what threat is seen

15. The mother of a client asks the nurse if obsessive-compulsive disorder and obsessive-compulsive personality disorder are the same disorder. Which of the following responses is the most appropriate?

    1. "A client with obsessive-compulsive personality disorder has an intense fear of self-contamination."

    2. "A client with obsessive-compulsive disorder is generally psychologically normal except in situations that evoke the obsession."

    3. "Obsessive-compulsive personality disorder can develop at any time during the client's lifetime."

    4. "A client with obsessive-compulsive disorder becomes extremely uncomfortable if anything in the surroundings gets moved."

16. A client with a diagnosis of histrionic personality disorder has a nursing diagnosis of

    1. Ineffective denial.

    2. Anxiety.

    3. Chronic low self-esteem.

    4. Impaired social interaction.

17. A nursing student asks the nurse if having a "hand-washing compulsion" while in the clinical area is a clinical manifestation of obsessive-compulsive personality disorder. The most appropriate response by the nurse is which of the following?

    1. "I think you should discuss your concerns with your doctor."

    2. "I don't think you have anything to worry about."

    3. "A persistent behavior is not a problem unless it leads to distress in your life."

    4. "Hand washing is a clinical manifestation of obsessive-compulsive personality disorder."

18. The nurse is teaching a class on the differences between schizophrenia, schizoid personality disorder, and schizotypal personality disorder. Which of the following statements should the nurse include in the class?

1. Clients with schizotypal personality disorder do not have ideas of reference and paranoia common in schizophrenia
2. The onset of schizophrenia can be traced to young adulthood or childhood
3. Only schizophrenia has the classic features of marked detachment, odd behavior, and social dysfunction
4. A client with schizoid or schizotypal personality disorder may go on to develop schizophrenia

19. The nurse is evaluating the following four clients for odd and eccentric behavior. Which of the following clients should the nurse suspect is experiencing a personality disorder?

1. A 44-year-old client who becomes very upset when anything in the environment becomes disarranged
2. An 86-year-old client who thinks she has been working at a clothing store in another state all day
3. A 14-year-old adolescent who suddenly is beginning to have trouble in school and has failing grades
4. A 51-year-old client who has paranoid beliefs that manifest themselves as delusions or hallucinations

20. The nurse is caring for a client who is very uncomfortable in situations in which the client is not the center of attention. The client dresses provocatively and has rapid shifts of emotion. Which of the following nursing diagnoses would be most appropriate?

1. Chronic low self-esteem
2. Ineffective denial
3. Impaired social interaction
4. Self-mutilation

21. Which of the following is a priority for the nurse to monitor for a client with borderline personality disorder?

1. Chronic feelings of emptiness
2. Transient, stress-related paranoid ideation
3. Self-mutilation
4. Inappropriate anger

22. The registered nurse is delegating nursing tasks to members of the health care team on a psychiatric unit. Which of the following tasks would be an appropriate delegation?

    1. Unlicensed assistive personnel walk clients to group therapy

    2. A licensed practical nurse develops the plan of care for a client with obsessive-compulsive personality disorder

    3. Unlicensed assistive personnel encourage clients to verbalize feelings

    4. A licensed practical nurse teaches a class on personality disorders

ANSWERS AND RATIONALES

1. **2, ,4 5.** A client with histrionic personality disorder constantly seeks attention through an excess of emotional expression. Such a client has an impressionistic style of speech, rapid shifts of emotions, considers relationships to be more intimate than they really are, and displays inappropriate sexually seductive or provocative behavior.
   NP = As
   CN = Ps/4
   CL = Ap
   SA = 2

2. **4.** Lack of empathy, being conceited, and feeling as though one is superior to others are indicative of narcissistic personality disorder. Clients with histrionic personality disorders do not lack empathy, and their need for attention is not filled by belittling other people, as it is with narcissistic personality disorder. Clients with borderline personality disorders have an emptiness and low self-worth, and therefore would not speak highly of themselves. Clients with avoidant personality disorder would not want to draw attention to themselves.
   NP = An
   CN = Ps/4
   CL = An
   SA = 2

3. **1, 2, 5.** A client with antisocial personality disorder focuses on a disregard of the law, impulsiveness, and a lack of remorse. A client with narcissistic personality disorder requires constant admiration. Exaggerated emotions and concern for physical appearance to draw attention to oneself are characteristics of histrionic personality disorder.
   NP = An
   CN = Ps/4
   CL = Ap
   SA = 2

4. 4. Classic features of avoidant personality disorder are social inhibition and feelings of inadequacy. Because of these characteristics, clients with avoidant personality disorder have an intense fear of doing new things. A lack of empathy is a clinical manifestation of narcissistic personality disorder. A client with schizoid personality has a lack of interest in pleasurable activities. A client who has paranoid personality disorder has a fear of being someone's target.
NP = Ev
CN = Ps/4
CL = An
SA = 2

5. 2. Avoidant personality is a disorder that exhibits a pattern of social inhibition, hypersensitivity to negativity, and feelings of inadequacy. When planning the care of a client with avoidant personality disorder, the nurse must consider the client's intense fear of rejection. Such clients are unwilling to get involved with an individual because they fear they will not be liked. A client who will likely let others assume responsibility is one who has dependent personality disorder. A client who does not desire a relationship with the nurse is one with schizoid personality disorder. Perceiving a situation as a threat is a clinical manifestation of a client with paranoid personality disorder.
NP = An
CN = Ps/4
CL = An
SA = 2

6. 3. A client with avoidant personality disorder is afraid of rejection, and engaging the client in interactions would be frightening. Such clients would not seek opportunities to interact. They also do not see their thoughts and fears as irrational and will need help to determine what fears are reality based. Bringing the client to a therapeutic group, challenging irrational thoughts, providing the opportunity for the client to seek out the nurse, and supporting the client's reluctance to engage in self-determination are all efforts to engage and would be detrimental to this client.
NP = Pl
CN = Ps/4
CL = Ap
SA = 2

7. dependent personality disorder. A client with borderline personality disorder displays instability in interpersonal relationships, self-image, and a pronounced impulsivity. Clients with borderline personality disorder do not directly seek reassurance but get reassurance from the chaos caused by

their erratic behavior. A tolerance for emotional, physical, or sexual abuse and self-sacrifice are the most striking features of dependent personality disorder when alternatives to self-care exist.

NP = An
CN = Ps/4
CL = An
SA = 2

8. **Obsessive-compulsive disorder.** Clients with obsessive-compulsive disorder are excessively preoccupied with order, cleanliness, control, and perfection. With obsessive-compulsive personality disorder, the client is comfortable with rituals and loses that comfort when things are not in order. Clients with obsessive-compulsive disorder are uncomfortable without their rituals. Behaviors such as checking doors and not stepping on cracks are examples of obsessive-compulsive behaviors.

NP = An
CN = Ps/4
CL = An
SA = 2

9. **4.** The behavior of a client with paranoid personality disorder is considered unpleasant but not bizarre or irrational. Hallucinations are generally absent. A client with paranoid schizophrenia often appears relatively normal before the onset of the illness. A client with paranoid personality disorder can often trace the illness to adolescence or even childhood. Characteristics such as distrust and suspicion are common in both illnesses.

NP = An
CN = Ps/4
CL = An
SA = 2

10. **1.** An extreme characteristic of grandiosity, lack of empathy, and a great need for admiration is present in narcissistic personality disorder. Engaging, listening, and connecting with the client who has narcissistic personality disorder will build rapport. The nurse should never encourage the grandiosity but must remain nonjudgmental to what the client says. Approaching the client in a cold, technical manner will stop the grandiosity but will also cause the therapeutic relationship to deteriorate.

NP = Pl
CN = Ps/4
CL = Ap
SA = 2

11. **4.** A client with avoidant personality disorder may never feel comfortable enough without encouragement to join the group. Remaining isolated will

foster the avoidance behaviors. The client needs to be encouraged to participate while acknowledging vulnerability. Therefore, any successes and accomplishments should be praised. Goal setting should be a combined effort of the nurse and client. The nurse needs to drive the advancement of the goals for the client to make progress.

NP = Pl
CN = Ps/4
CL = Ap
SA = 2

12. 2. A client with obsessive-compulsive personality disorder does not like to relinquish control for fear something may go wrong. The constant drive for perfection leads to indecisiveness because of the fear of making the wrong decision. Although preoccupation with details and reluctance to delegate are important characteristics of obsessive-compulsive disorder, the client's indecisiveness is the priority. It is the indecisiveness that leads to the other clinical manifestations, such as the client's preoccupation with details and reluctance to delegate tasks. Such clients are not envious of others; in fact, they often pity others for not being more like themselves.

NP = An
CN = Sa/1
CL = An
SA = 2

13. 3. Task completion that is hampered by the client's desire for perfection is a classic feature in obsessive-compulsive personality disorder. Clients with narcissistic personality disorder are focused on their fantasies of unlimited success. Clients with paranoid personality disorder look for hidden meanings in the actions of others. Although clients with dependent personality disorder have trouble with task completion, theirs is the result of a lack of confidence.

NP = An
CN = Ps/4
CL = An
SA = 2

14. 1. A client with dependent personality disorder is eager to start any kind of relationship. Such a client will go anywhere at any time for the sense of attachment and security. Clients eager to be admired are representative of narcissistic personality disorder. The vacillation between wanting a relationship and then pushing it away is indicative of borderline personality disorder.

NP = An
CN = Ps/4
CL = An
SA = 2

15. 2. A client with obsessive-compulsive disorder may appear psychologically normal except in situations that cause the obsession or compulsion. Such clients have an intense fear of becoming self-contaminated, resulting in a ritualistic type of hand-washing behavior. The obsessive-compulsive disorder can begin at any time during the individual's life. In contrast, obsessive-compulsive personality disorder generally begins in young adulthood or childhood. A client with obsessive-compulsive personality disorder becomes very uncomfortable if anything in the surroundings is moved.
NP = An
CN = Ps/4
CL = An
SA = 2

16. 4. Appropriate nursing diagnoses for clients with a diagnosis of histrionic personality disorder is impaired social interaction and ineffective coping. A nursing diagnosis of Ineffective denial would be common in narcissistic and antisocial personality disorders. Anxiety would be a nursing diagnosis in paranoid and obsessive-compulsive personality disorders. Chronic low self-esteem is a nursing diagnosis common in borderline, obsessive-compulsive, and dependent personality disorders.
NP = Ev
CN = Ps/4
CL = An
SA = 2

17. 3. It is normal for a nursing student to identify with clinical manifestations of diseases they are studying in class. Hand washing is particularly stressed in schools of nursing as an important nursing task in the prevention of infection. It is actually the first line of defense in the prevention of spreading infection. An activity or behavior, such as hand washing, does not become a problem unless it causes great distress in the individual's life.
NP = An
CN = Ps/4
CL = An
SA = 2

18. 4. Clients with schizotypal personality disorder have ideas of reference and paranoia common in schizophrenia. The difference is they are less intense in the schizotypal personality disorder. Clients with schizophrenia have normal personalities before becoming ill. It is only after the onset that they have a serious cognitive and social impairment. The classic features of marked detachment, odd behavior, and social dysfunction are present in schizophrenia, schizoid personality disorder, and schizotypal personality disorder.

NP = An
CN = Ps/4
CL = An
SA = 2

19. 3. A 44-year-old client who becomes very upset when anything in the environment becomes disarranged is displaying a clinical manifestation of obsessive-compulsive disorder. An 86-year-old client who thinks she has been working all day in a clothing store in another state is exhibiting dementia. A 51-year-old client who has paranoid beliefs that manifest themselves as delusions or hallucinations is exhibiting a feature of paranoid schizophrenia. Paranoid beliefs in paranoid personality disorder are more unpleasant than irrational and bizarre. Delusions and hallucinations are absent. Personality disorders can be traced to young adulthood or childhood. A 14-year-old client who is beginning to have trouble in school or failing grades may be experiencing the onset of a personality disorder.
NP = Ev
CN = Ps/4
CL = An
SA = 2

20. 3. A client who is uncomfortable in situations when not the center of attention, has rapid shifts of emotion, and dresses provocatively has histrionic personality disorder. The most appropriate nursing diagnosis is Impaired social interaction. A nursing diagnosis of Chronic low self-esteem is appropriate for a client with borderline, obsessive-compulsive, or dependent personality disorders. Ineffective denial is an effective nursing diagnosis for narcissistic and antisocial personality disorders. Self-mutilation is an appropriate nursing diagnosis for a client with borderline personality disorder.
NP = An
CN = Ps/4
CL = An
SA = 2

21. 3. Although clients with borderline personality disorder have chronic feelings of emptiness, transient and stress-related paranoid ideation, and inappropriate anger, the priority for this client is to monitor for self-mutilation. These clients have recurrent suicidal behaviors, gestures, or self-mutilating behavior.
NP = As
CN = Ps/4
CL = An
SA = 2

22. **1.** It would be appropriate to delegate walking a client to group therapy as a task for unlicensed assistive personnel. Unlicensed personnel should not be encouraging a client to verbalize feelings. Teaching a class and developing a plan of care are tasks that should be performed by a registered nurse.
NP = Pl
CN = Sa/1
CL = An
SA = 8

MOOD DISORDERS - COMPREHENSIVE EXAM

1. A client who had one depressive episode asks the nurse if future depressive episodes will be experienced. The most appropriate response by the nurse is

    1. "Individuals who become depressed will have depression most of one's life."

    2. "If you have had one depressive episode, you have a 60% chance of having another."

    3. "Depression is situational and you most likely will never have another episode."

    4. "You have a 70% chance of getting depressed at some point in your life."

2. Based on an understanding of medical terminology, what is the appropriate term the nurse should use to document when a client with major depression has fatigue and a loss of energy? _____

3. The nurse assesses which of the following clinical manifestations to be present in a client suspected of having major depression?
Select all that apply:
    [ ] **1.** Flight of ideas
    [ ] **2.** Anhedonia
    [ ] **3.** Indecisiveness
    [ ] **4.** Talkativeness
    [ ] **5.** Hypersomnia
    [ ] **6.** Grandiosity

4. The nurse is admitting a client with mania and a nursing diagnosis of Imbalanced nutrition: less than body requirements as evidenced by

reported inadequate food intake. When intervening in this situation, the nurse should

Select all that apply:

[   ] 1. offer three well-balanced meals per day

[   ] 2. provide the client with high-calorie snacks

[   ] 3. arrange for "finger foods" to be brought to the client

[   ] 4. offer food every 15 minutes

[   ] 5. encourage the client to avoid activities

[   ] 6. offer the client juice and cold beverages

5. Because a client has a bipolar mood disorder, the priority nursing intervention includes

1. family history.

2. current mood assessment.

3. evaluation of attention span.

4. assessment of intellectual functioning.

6. Which of the following is a priority nursing intervention when planning the care for a hospitalized client who has bipolar I disorder and is exhibiting clinical manifestations of grandiosity, impulsiveness, and flight of ideas?

1. Encourage adequate nutrition

2. Initiate the discharge process

3. Decrease stimuli within the environment

4. Promote safety for the client and others

7. When developing the outcome criteria for a client in an outpatient setting who has major depression and is at risk for a self-inflicted, life-threatening injury, the priority nursing intervention is to

1. demonstrate use of alternative ways of managing stress and emotional issues.

2. avoid harming self or others.

3. verbalize plans for continuing outpatient therapy.

4. demonstrate use of the problem-solving process.

8. The nurse is admitting a client who is suicidal to an inpatient psychiatric unit. In this situation, the priority nursing intervention would be for the nurse to

1. explore grief and loss issues with the client.

2. ensure that the client is not permitted to use anything that would be potentially dangerous.

 3. encourage the client to express feelings of anger.

 4. explore with the client ways to recognize and manage suicidal thoughts.

9. Which of the following is most appropriate for the nurse to include when preparing to teach a class on bipolar disorders?

 1. The client alternates between mania and hypomania behavior at the same time

 2. The hypomania episode comes first and is followed by a manic episode

 3. The clinical manifestations of hypomania behavior are different from mania

 4. With the progression of the clinical course, the client goes from sociability and euphoria to hostility, irritability, and paranoia

10. Which of the following nursing responses would be most therapeutic when working with a client in a manic state?

 1. "Don't worry, you'll come out of this soon."

 2. "The best part of the illness is the manic state because you have so much energy."

 3. "I notice you have a high energy level. What are some things that have helped you to relax in the past?"

 4. "Your manic states usually last about 4 to 5 days. In 5 days, we can discuss treatment options."

11. A hospitalized client with major depression has been referred to a therapist for psychotherapy. The client asks the nurse what the benefit is for receiving psychotherapy. The most appropriate response by the nurse would be

 1. "Psychotherapy provides emotional support and provides an opportunity for self-awareness."

 2. "Psychotherapy prevents clients from becoming depressed."

 3. "Psychotherapy ensures that total recovery from the major depressive episode will occur."

 4. "Psychotherapy offers the client respite from stressful situations."

12. When planning care for a client with dysthymia, which of the following cognitive or behavioral nursing interventions should the nurse include?

 1. Advise that a negative view of life can be a self-fulfilling prophecy

 2. Administer phototherapy

 3. Conduct a comprehensive physical exam

 4. Administer a healthy diet

13. Which of the following subjective information should the nurse obtain when assessing a client for schizoaffective disorder?

    1. Affect and global assessment of functioning

    2. Presence of hallucinations

    3. Appearance and hygiene

    4. Weight and level of activity

14. The nurse is collecting data on a cyclothymic mood disorder. Which of the following assessment information is a priority to obtain?

    1. Mood changes

    2. Family history

    3. Recent food intake

    4. Appearance and hygiene

15. Which of the following should the nurse consider when planning the care of a client with a bipolar disorder?
    Select all that apply:

    [ ] 1. Occurs more commonly in middle-age women

    [ ] 2. Stressful life events contribute to the onset

    [ ] 3. Hypochondriasis, insomnia, and increased motor activity are clinical manifestations

    [ ] 4. Has a high sense of guilt

    [ ] 5. Has a high frequency of relapse

    [ ] 6. There is a greater risk in the suburbs

16. When assessing a client for a substance-induced mood disorder, the most accurate information the nurse would need to assess would be

    1. identifying any recent physical injuries that have occurred within 1 month of substance intoxication or withdrawal.

    2. identifying the season of the year that the client has the most difficulty with substance use and difficulty with mood.

    3. confirming that mood manifestations have occurred within 1 month of substance intoxication or withdrawal.

    4. identifying if the client has increased or decreased sexual activity within periods of substance use.

17. Ongoing nursing care measures associated with depression should include

    1. provide instruction regarding diet and its effect on mood.

    2. instruct the client about the possibility of manic episodes.

    3. educate the client about need for electroconvulsive therapy.

    4. encourage rest and time spent alone.

18. A client comes to the emergency room complaining of depression. Which of the following criteria most appropriately indicates that the client needs to be admitted to the hospital?

    1. The client reports having thoughts of suicide, with no plan and a minimal support system available at home

    2. The client verbalizes no hope for the future, and has had a poor appetite for a number of weeks

    3. The client expresses the need to cry and a sleep disturbance

    4. The client complains of decreased libido and decreased energy

19. While providing education to a client recovering from depression, the nurse recognizes that the most effective prevention of recurrent depression is for the client to

    1. obtain frequent electroconvulsive therapy.

    2. concurrently use an antidepressant drug and psychotherapy.

    3. reduce weight and participate in an exercise program.

    4. abstain from alcohol.

20. The nurse is planning the care of a client with bipolar depression. Which of the following measures would be essential to include in the care of the client experiencing hypomania?

    1. Encourage unsupervised activities

    2. Give direct, clear responses to the client

    3. Explore triggers that precipitate episodes of hypomania

    4. Explain systematic desensitization to the client

21. The nurse is caring for a client with schizoaffective disorder who is currently experiencing auditory and visual hallucinations. Which of the following nursing measures should receive priority in the client's plan of care?

    1. Engage the client in reality-based conversation

    2. Recognize the strengths and accomplishments of the client

    3. Encourage the client to participate in one-to-one activities

    4. Discuss with the client how to prevent a relapse

22. A client is admitted to the hospital with major depression. Which of the following is a priority behavior necessitating that the client be placed on constant observation by a staff member?

    1. The client is smoking on the unit in which there is no smoking allowed

    2. The client is agitated and calling names to other clients

    3. The client is unable to assure the staff that no self-harm will occur

    4. The client is exhibiting paranoia and attempting to hit staff during care

23. What assessment exam is a priority for the nurse to perform on a client suspected of having a mood disorder? _____

24. The nurse is gathering information on the health history form for a client recently admitted for a sleep disturbance and a possible diagnosis of dysthymia. Which of the following questions would be the priority for the nurse to ask to substantiate a diagnosis of dysthymia?

    1. "How long have you been experiencing difficulty with low self-esteem and depression?"

    2. "How long have you had trouble sleeping?"

    3. "Do you have any problems with your appetite?"

    4. "Are you feeling hopeless?"

25. The nurse is caring for a client with a major depressive disorder. Which of the following observations should the nurse report immediately? Select all that apply:

    [ ] 1. Insomnia

    [ ] 2. Poor fluid intake

    [ ] 3. Hopelessness

    [ ] 4. Decreased libido

    [ ] 5. Passive death wish

    [ ] 6. Low self-esteem

26. The registered nurse is preparing to delegate nursing tasks on a psychiatric unit. Which of the following tasks should the nurse delegate to a licensed practical nurse?

    1. Develop a teaching plan for a client with depression who is on a diet

    2. Develop a medication schedule for a client with depression

    3. Instruct a client with depression on the importance of combined drug and psychotherapy

    4. Encourage a client with depression to participate in group therapy

ANSWERS AND RATIONALES

1. **2.** If an individual has one depressive episode, there is a 60% chance of getting a second episode of depression. If an individual has a second depressive episode, there is a 70% chance of getting a third episode. Individuals who have a third episode of depression have a 90% chance of getting future episodes.
   NP = An
   CN = Ps/4

CL = An
SA = 2

2. **Anergia.** Anergia is the term for fatigue and loss of energy associated with a major depressive episode.
NP = Im
CN = Ps/4
CL = Co
SA = 2

3. **2, 3, 6.** The diagnostic criteria for a major depressive episode includes at least five of the following clinical manifestations every day for a period of 2 weeks or more: depressive mood, anhedonia, anergia, weight loss or gain, self-worthlessness, guilt, indecisiveness, decreased concentration, insomnia, hypersomnia, decreased or increased activity level, and a predisposition to suicidal thoughts. A client who has flight of ideas, talkativeness, and grandiosity meets the criteria for a diagnosis of a bipolar disorder.
NP = As
CN = Ps/4
CL = Ap
SA = 2

4. **3, 4, 6.** The most appropriate interventions for a client who has a medical diagnosis of mania and a nursing diagnosis of Imbalanced nutrition: less than body requirements, as evidenced by reported inadequate food intake, include offering food every 15 minutes for the first hour after admission to the unit. The nurse should offer cold beverages, water, juices, and "finger foods," such as sandwiches, crackers, and fruit. Implementing these interventions facilitate the nursing outcome that the client will eat some food and become well hydrated.
NP = Im
CN = Ps/4
CL = Ap
SA = 2

5. **2.** Clients with a bipolar mood disorder have varying levels of mood, which go from high levels of mood (mania) to low levels of mood (depression). An assessment of the client's current mood is a priority assessment. This ensures that all subsequent interventions are appropriate for the client's current status.
NP = Pl
CN = Sa/1
CL = Ap
SA = 2

6. 4. The priority nursing intervention for a client who has bipolar I disorder and is experiencing grandiosity, impulsiveness, and flight of ideas is to ensure safety for the client and others. Bipolar I disorder is the classic manic-depressive disease with a combination of depression and at least one episode of mania.
NP = Pl
CN = Sa/1
CL = Ap
SA = 8

7. 2. Because there is such a high risk of self-inflicted harm to a client with major depression, the priority intervention is to prevent the client from harming oneself and others. Demonstrating alternative ways of managing stress and emotional issues, verbalizing plans for continuing outpatient therapy, and demonstrating the use of problem-solving techniques are all appropriate interventions but not the priority.
NP = Pl
CN = Sa/1
CL = An
SA = 8

8. 2. Although exploring grief and loss issues, encouraging the client to explore feelings of anger, and exploring with the client ways to recognize and manage suicidal thoughts are all important interventions, the priority intervention for a client who is suicidal is to ensure that the client is not permitted to use anything that would be considered potentially dangerous.
NP = Pl
CN = Sa/1
CL = An
SA = 8

9. 4. Although a client may experience episodes of mania and hypomania at the same time, generally the two conditions are experienced separately. Usually the manic behavior comes first, followed by the hypomanic behavior. The diagnostic criteria for hypomania and mania are very similar. To meet the criteria for hypomania, the client must have at least four of the seven classic manifestations. As the clinical course, or switch from hypomania to mania, progresses, the client goes from sociability and euphoria to hostility, irritability, and paranoia.
NP = Pl
CN = Ps/4
CL = Ap
SA = 2

10. 3. Recognizing the client's high energy level first, followed by asking the client what kinds of things helped the client to relax in the past, is the therapeutic response for a client in a manic state. It would not be therapeutic to tell the client not to worry because the manic state will end. Nor is it therapeutic to tell the client that the mania is the best part of the illness or to postpone discussing treatment options.
NP = An
CN = Ps/4
CL = An
SA = 2

11. 1. Psychotherapy alone may not prevent the client from becoming depressed in the future. Psychotherapy does not ensure that total recovery from major depression is inevitable. Psychotherapy addresses emotional issues and provides an avenue to discuss ways to more effectively manage stressful situations, rather than providing respite from stressful situations.
NP = An
CN = Ps/4
CL = An
SA = 2

12. 1. Cognitive or behavioral therapy assists the client in becoming more aware of one's own thoughts, feelings, and subsequent actions or behaviors in response to upsetting situations. Cognitive therapy also addresses how one's unrealistic or negative view of life can become a self-fulfilling prophecy.
NP = Pl
CN = Ps/4
CL = Ap
SA = 2

13. 2. Assessing for the presence of hallucinations is a subjective datum because the client would have to verbalize what is being seen. The client's claim that hallucinations are present in a client experiencing a schizoaffective disorder cannot be measured and so is not objective. Assessments of functioning, appearance, hygiene, weight, and level of activity are all objective data.
NP = As
CN = Ps/4
CL = Ap
SA = 2

14. 1. It is most important to assess mood states and the presence of rapid, abrupt mood changes in a client with a cyclothymic disorder. Obtaining a family history, recent food intake, appearance, and hygiene are additional

interventions that may be appropriate, but these are not the priority. Cyclothymic disorder is a mood disturbance of at least a 2-year duration that involves both hypomania and dysthymic mood swings.

NP = As
CN = Sa/1
CL = Ap
SA = 2

15. 2, 5, 6. Bipolar disorders occur most commonly in individuals between the ages of 19 and 30 years of age living in the suburbs. Clinical manifestations include psychomotor retardation, hypersomnia, and minimal anxiety. There are also traits of dominance, exhibition, and autonomy present. There is a greater risk in the suburbs.

NP = Pl
CN = Ps/4
CL = Ap
SA = 2

16. 3. When assessing a client for a substance-induced mood disorder, the most accurate information is to confirm that the mood manifestations have occurred within 1 month of substance intoxication or withdrawal. Physical injuries will not give the nurse the information to determine if the mood disorder is caused by a mood-altering substance. It is important to assess the season of the year that may be most difficult for the client, but this information will not ensure that it is a substance-induced mood disorder. Sexual activity will not give the necessary information needed to confirm a diagnosis of a substance-induced mood disorder.

NP = As
CN = Ps/4
CL = Ap
SA = 2

17. 1. The client with depression is encouraged to get approximately 8 hours of sleep but needs to spend time around others to decrease the sense of isolation. Depression is not synonymous with mania. Many clients can be successfully treated with antidepressants and psychotherapy and would not need electroconvulsive therapy. The nurse may plan care for the client who is depressed by providing instruction on a variety of foods in the diet that can assist with elevating one's mood.

NP = Pl
CN = Ps/4
CL = Ap
SA = 2

18. 2. If a client has an adequate support system available at home, the family and friends can be called to assist with monitoring the client at the home,

with an outpatient follow-up. Complaints of frequent crying and sleep disturbance and complaints of decreased libido and energy are not sufficient to warrant hospitalization. A client who reports that there is no hope for the future and has not been eating for several weeks is at a greater risk for suicide and requires hospitalization.
NP = Ev
CN = Ps/4
CL = Ap
SA = 2

19. 2. Research has found that clients with depression do best when taking an antidepressant drug along with attending psychotherapy. If an individual discontinues the antidepressant drug and depression recurs within several months, the individual will need to continue on the antidepressant drug to prevent recurrent depressive episodes.
NP = An
CN = Ps/4
CL = An
SA = 2

20. 2. The client with hypomania needs to be observed in structured activities to provide safety for the client. Providing structure also teaches the client to have appropriate boundaries. Exploring triggers that precipitate episodes of hypomania may be difficult for the client with hypomanic clinical manifestations, due to the client's high energy level and decreased insight into behavior. Systematic desensitization is not a treatment of choice for the client with hypomania. It is most appropriate to give the client clear, direct responses in the plan of care, because they provide consistent feedback to the client who is exhibiting erratic behavior.
NP = Pl
CN = Ps/4
CL = Ap
SA = 2

21. 1. Although recognizing the strengths and accomplishments of the client, encouraging the client to participate in one-to-one activities, and discussing with the client ways to prevent a relapse are important interventions in the care of the client with schizoaffective disorder, engaging the client in reality-based conversation is a priority.
NP = Pl
CN = Sa/1
CL = An
SA = 8

22. 3. The behavior of a client who is smoking in a no smoking area should be dealt with. Cigarettes and matches can be taken away from the client. A client who is agitated and calling names to other clients should be placed in a less stimulating environment. When a client is paranoid and hitting staff, the staff can leave the client alone until the client is more approachable. Clients who are unable to verbally contract with a staff member that they will not harm themselves are at risk for self-directed violence and should be the priority for continual observation by a staff member.
NP = Ev
CN = Sa/1
CL = An
SA = 8

23. Mental status exam. A mental status exam is necessary when assessing a client with a mood disorder. The mental status exam includes gathering information regarding an individual's mood, affect, sensorium, orientation, along with completing a suicide assessment.
NP = As
CN = Sa/1
CL = Ap
SA = 2

24. 1. Assessing for sleep and appetite disturbances along with feelings of hopelessness are important in the assessment of the client for dysthymia. However, asking the client if there are long-standing issues of low self-esteem along with a depressed mood is the priority to substantiate a mood disorder such as dysthymia, since it is a chronic low mood.
NP = An
CN = Sa/1
CL = An
SA = 2

25. 2, 3 5. Initially, insomnia is more likely to be seen in a client who is anxious rather than depressed. Also, low self-esteem and decreased libido are not needed to be reported immediately. Poor fluid intake and poor nutritional intake can result in dehydration, nutritional imbalances, and fluid and electrolyte imbalances, so they should be reported. Feelings of hopelessness and a passive death wish are extremely important to report, because the client would most likely be on constant observation to protect the client from self-directed violence and suicide. This is an issue of safety.
NP = An
CN = Ps/4
CL = An
SA = 2

26. 4. A licensed practical nurse may encourage a client to participate in group therapy. Developing a teaching plan and medication schedule and instructing a client are tasks that are reserved for the registered nurse.

NP = Pl
CN = Sa/1
CL = An
SA = 8

SCHIZOPHRENIA AND PSYCHOTIC DISORDERS - COMPREHENSIVE EXAM

1. The nurse evaluates a client who is having trouble completing a sentence before quickly moving on to the next topic and sentence. What is the client experiencing? _____

2. A client with schizophrenia becomes loud and threatening in the dining room. Which of the following is the priority nursing intervention?
   1. Obtain help to escort the client to seclusion
   2. Instruct the client to calm down
   3. Ask the other clients to relocate
   4. Avoid the client to see if the behavior stops

3. A client states, "I can hear the other clients talking about me and laughing." The most appropriate nursing response is
   1. "You must be hearing voices again."
   2. "What are they saying?"
   3. "You must feel terrible when you hear that."
   4. "I'm sorry, I don't hear any voices."

4. A male client has a history of delusions involving the belief that he has been appointed to bring all the world countries to peace. The girlfriend confirms this and believes that this is his role in the world. The nurse identifies this as _____.

5. A client who has schizophrenia is admitted to the inpatient psychiatric unit. The client is actively hallucinating and is unable to provide information for the admission process. What is the nurse's best option for getting information?
   1. Wait until the medication works
   2. Ask the next shift to do the admission
   3. Get the information from the physician
   4. Ask the client's family for information

6. A client with the diagnosis of schizophrenia has been assigned a nurse case manager. The primary nursing diagnosis for this client is Thought processes, disturbed. Which of the following would be the nursing outcome for this client?

   1. The client is rehospitalized
   2. The client's family is more involved
   3. The client reports a decreased number of hallucinations
   4. The client reports taking medication only when needed

7. In planning the care of a client experiencing paranoid delusions, which of the following is the priority goal?

   1. Absence of delusions
   2. Establishing trust
   3. Participation in all unit activities
   4. Performing independent activities

8. A client who is diagnosed with schizophrenia is preparing for discharge by reviewing relapse prevention with the nurse. The client states an understanding of when to seek help with which of the following?

   1. Reporting that a part-time job is in place when discharged
   2. Understanding stressful situations that precipitated past psychotic episodes
   3. Describing the uses and schedule for drugs
   4. Requesting the home phone numbers of physicians and therapists

9. The nurse caring for a client with schizophrenia should monitor the client for which of the following positive manifestations?
   Select all that apply:

   [   ] 1. Disorganized speech
   [   ] 2. Avolition
   [   ] 3. Hallucination
   [   ] 4. Flat affect
   [   ] 5. Delusions
   [   ] 6. Anhedonia

10. The nurse should administer what classification of drugs to a client who has a delusional disorder and fears being captured by the Central Intelligence Agency (CIA)? _____

11. The nurse should monitor a client who was admitted with catatonic schizophrenia for which of the following?

   1. Nonstop talk about a number of different topics
   2. Unusual body postures displayed

3. Thoughts of having an undiagnosed cancer

4. Self-identification as Jesus Christ

12. A client diagnosed with chronic disorganized schizophrenia has been through the inpatient psychiatric program three times prior to the current hospitalization. Upon discharge, the nurse makes contact with the client's community mental health nurse case manager. The nurse understands that the priority goal of the nurse case manager is to

1. provide social contact.

2. decrease recidivism.

3. get medication for the client.

4. increase the client's safety.

13. Which of the following indicates that the public health nurse needs to provide more social skills enhancement measures for the client with a psychotic disorder? The client demonstrates

1. attendance at a consumer warehouse club.

2. interest in getting a job.

3. conflict resolution with family members.

4. frequent, insignificant calls to the public health nurse.

14. The nurse evaluates which of the following comments by a client with a delusional disorder as indicating the client has made improvement?

1. "Dr. Jones is in love with me."

2. "My spouse is having an affair."

3. "I don't have any signs of cancer."

4. "The Federal Bureau of Investigation is watching my house."

15. Which of the following comments by a client indicate the need for an urgent dose of an antipsychotic drug?

1. "The voices are mumbling and I can't hear them very well."

2. "The voices are telling me to rip my bed sheet and hang myself."

3. "The voice I heard this morning sounded like my dead grandmother."

4. "The voices told me to kill my neighbor when I get home."

16. Which of the following is the most plausible explanation a client's family gives the nurse that the client's brief psychotic episode was normal?

1. It is accepted within their religion

2. The client is a drug addict

3. The client has an infection

4. It has happened only once before

17. A client who experiences chronic auditory hallucinations is learning how to cope with them. What is the best advice the nurse can give to the client for coping enhancement?

    1. "Focus on internal feelings."
    2. "Daydream when you feel lonely."
    3. "Stick to a structured schedule."
    4. "Talk back to the voices."

18. A client admits to the nurse of hearing voices giving directions to talk to the doctor immediately. When the nurse inquires why, the client won't say. What is the nurse's first intervention?

    1. Try to convince the client that the voices are not real
    2. Assess the effect of the voices on the doctor's safety
    3. Allow the client free time to make a choice of activity
    4. Get the restraints and seclusion area ready

19. A client has recovered from an acute episode of schizophrenia but continues with a lack of energy and decreased interest in activities. What is the best nursing diagnosis for this client's current situation?

    1. Thought processes, disturbed
    2. Role performance, ineffective
    3. Risk for violence
    4. Health maintenance, ineffective

20. A client whose psychotic clinical manifestations are well controlled by antipsychotics is NPO pending a diagnostic test. The nurse should monitor the client for which of the following after the client misses one dose of the antipsychotic drug?

    1. Disorganized thinking
    2. Daytime somnolence
    3. Aggressive behavior
    4. Suicidal thoughts

21. A client on the inpatient unit is hearing a group of voices mumbling. The hallucinations are so distracting that the client cannot clearly hear the nurse speaking. What treatment intervention should the nurse implement at this point?

    1. Talk to the client in a louder tone of voice
    2. Distract the client with a unit activity
    3. Ask another nurse to talk to the client
    4. Assess the client in a quiet, nonstimulating area

22. The client with disorganized schizophrenia is having difficulty reentering previous community activities following a hospitalization discharge. The community nurse will help the client become reintegrated into the community by

   1. making extra home visits.
   2. convincing the client of self-worth.
   3. teaching specific social skills.
   4. pointing out grooming deficits.

23. A client who is diagnosed with residual schizophrenia lacks motivation to complete self-directed activities. While observing the client this would be evident by the client

   1. dressing in mismatched clothing.
   2. having a cold breakfast instead of hot.
   3. having an inability to complete adequate hygiene.
   4. exhibiting a sense of tiredness on awakening.

24. A client reports having just seen Saddam Hussein and tells the nurse that Saddam is on the unit. The nurse's best response would be

   1. "I know you believe that, but he's not here."
   2. "You are definitely hallucinating again."
   3. "That's ridiculous! He could never get on the unit."
   4. "Where did you see him?"

25. A client is sentenced to 3 days in jail for driving while intoxicated. Toward the end of the stay, the client tells the jail officer of hearing voices. The nurse reports this as most likely due to

   1. first onset schizophrenia-related psychosis.
   2. manipulation to get out of jail.
   3. delirium tremens related to alcohol withdrawal.
   4. residual effects of a head injury that occurred when the client was a child.

26. The registered nurse is preparing to make the clinical assignments on a psychiatric unit. Which of the following assignments should the nurse delegate to a licensed practical nurse?

   1. Monitor a client with schizophrenia for positive clinical manifestations
   2. Assess a client with schizophrenia for hallucinations
   3. Administer an antipsychotic drug to a client with schizophrenia
   4. Develop a plan of care for a client exhibiting schizophrenia

ANSWERS AND RATIONALES

1. **Flight of ideas.** Flight of ideas is a rapid succession of speech in which the client jumps from one topic to another. It is a classic feature in schizophrenia.
NP = An
CN = Ps/4
CL = Ap
SA = 2

2. 3. Asking the other clients to relocate after a client becomes loud and threatening in the dining room is the most appropriate intervention because safety is always the priority. Instructing the client to calm down would impede the client's desire to be heard. Escorting the client to seclusion is not the most appropriate intervention, because less restrictive interventions must be tried before seclusion. Waiting to see if the behavior stops is not appropriate, because the client is not likely to stop the behavior once it has already escalated to being loud and threatening.
NP = Pl
CN = Sa/1
CL = Ap
SA = 8

3. 4. An appropriate response to a client who verbalizes hearing other clients talk about the client is that the nurse does not hear the voices. This response provides reality orientation. It promotes honesty and trust in a client-provider relationship. Asking the client what the voices are saying allows the nurse to engage with the client about the misperceptions. Offering that the client must feel terrible when the client hears another client talk or acknowledging that the client must be hearing the voices again do not provide reality orientation for the client.
NP = An
CN = Ps/4
CL = An
SA = 2

4. **shared psychotic disorder.** A shared psychotic disorder is a situation that consists of an individual having a specific delusion with a second individual sharing that same delusion. The delusion is not erotic in nature. Delusions can occur without schizophrenia. Two individuals who have a shared belief are not the result of a cult.
NP = An
CN = Ps/4

CL = An
SA = 2

5. 4. Waiting until a drug works or asking the next shift to do the admission delays the gathering of information. Getting information from the physician is not appropriate because the nurse must do the admission. The most accurate and timely method of obtaining critical information is from the family.
NP = Im
CN = Ps/4
CL = An
SA = 2

6. 3. The most appropriate outcome is that the client reports having a decreased number of hallucinations. This outcome directly corresponds to altered thoughts, such as hallucinations. Rehospitalizing the client does not represent a positive goal with regard to thought disorders. Getting the client's family more involved does not directly relate to goals regarding an individual's thoughts. A client who reports taking a drug only when needed is taking an action related to medication compliance.
NP = Ev
CN = Ps/4
CL = An
SA = 2

7. 2. The priority goal when working with a client experiencing delusions is to establish a trusting relationship. It is only after establishing trust that the client will buy into the treatment plan and goals. Being absent of delusions, participating in all unit activities, and performing independent activities may be appropriate interventions but not the priorities.
NP = Ev
CN = Sa/1
CL = An
SA = 8

8. 2. A client who can verbalize the understanding that stressful situations precipitated past psychotic episodes recognizes that information and skills learned while in the hospital can be applied in a different situation. Requesting a part-time job after getting home from the hospital or describing the use and schedule of drugs represent adequate functioning. Requesting the home phone numbers of physicians and therapists represents a request that goes beyond healthy boundaries.
NP = Ev
CN = Ps/4
CL = An
SA = 2

9. 1, 3, 5. Three classic positive clinical manifestations of schizophrenia include disordered thought and behavior, hallucinations, and delusions. Unlike negative clinical manifestations, positive clinical manifestations appear bizarre even to individuals with no special training. They are easier to detect than negative manifestations. The negative manifestations of schizophrenia include flat affect, alogia (speaking and using brief and empty phrases), avolition (lack of motivation), anhedonia (inability to find pleasure in events or activities), and flat affect.
NP = As
CN = Ps/4
CL = Ap
SA = 2

10. **Antipsychotics.** Antipsychotics are the classification of drugs that are administered for thought disorders such as a fear of being captured by the CIA.
NP = Im
CN = Ps/4
CL = Ap
SA = 2

11. 2. Catatonia describes the motor activity of an individual with schizophrenia. It is a state of immobilization that has periods of severe agitation. A client who talks nonstop about a number of different topics is experiencing flight of ideas. Having a thought of an undiagnosed cancer is a somatic delusion. A client who self-identifies as Jesus Christ is exhibiting a grandiose delusion.
NP = As
CN = Ps/4
CL = An
SA = 2

12. 2. The primary goal of the case manager role is to decrease recidivism.
NP = Ev
CN = Sa/1
CL = An
SA = 8

13. 4. A client with a psychotic disorder who is making frequent, insignificant calls to the public health nurse is indicating that the client needs additional social skills enhancement measures. Attendance at a consumer warehouse club, interest in getting a job, and conflict resolution with family members are all indications of a higher level of social functioning.
NP = Ev
CN = Ps/4
CL = An
SA = 2

14. 3. A client with a delusional disorder who verbalizes that there are no signs of cancer is indicating that the client's disorder has improved. This demonstrates a lack of a somatic delusion. A client who says that a doctor is in love with the client is experiencing an erotomanic delusion. A client who verbalizes that a spouse having an affair is expressing a jealous delusion. A client who feels that the Federal Bureau of Investigation is watching the house indicates that the client is having a persecutory delusion.
NP = Ev
CN = Ps/4
CL = An
SA = 2

15. 2. A client who says voices are telling the client to rip a bed sheet and hang oneself indicates an urgent need for the administration of an antipsychotic drug. This comment indicates that the client is suicidal with a plan. Although a client who verbalizes wanting to kill a neighbor after being discharged from the hospital indicates a need for a drug to be administered, it is not an urgent need.
NP = Ev
CN = Ps/4
CL = An
SA = 2

16. 1. Some religions and cultures may accept some experiences, including seeing visions and hearing voices, as normal even though these manifestations may fit criteria for a psychotic episode.
NP = An
CN = Ps/4
CL = An
SA = 2

17. 3. Telling a client who is experiencing auditory hallucinations to focus on internal feelings, to daydream when feeling lonely, or to talk back to the voices are all counterproductive to providing diversion and coping methods. A structured schedule will provide the greatest chance for the client to remain functional even while experiencing a perceptual disturbance.
NP = An
CN = Ps/4
CL = An
SA = 2

18. 2. The most appropriate intervention to implement when a client reports hearing voices telling the client to see the doctor immediately is to assess the effect of the voices on the doctor's safety. Safety is always the priority

and may be an issue since the client is not forthcoming with why the physician needs to be seen. Trying to convince the client that the voices are not real contradicts this client's reality. Allowing the client free time to make a choice of activity does not provide enough structure for the client. Getting restraints and a seclusion area ready is not the least restrictive intervention. There is also no evidence at this point that the client's or other individual's safety is in jeopardy.
NP = Im
CN = Ps/4
CL = Ap
SA = 8

19. 2. Ineffective role performance is the most appropriate intervention for a client who has recovered from an acute episode of schizophrenia, because the lack of energy and decreased interest will mostly affect the client's ability to perform usual daily activities of living. Disturbed thought process and Risk for violence pertain to the client's thought processes. Ineffective health maintenance relates to the information the client understands about the diagnosis.
NP = An
CN = Ps/4
CL = An
SA = 2

20. 1. A single missed dose of an antipsychotic will decrease the client's serum level of the drug and may result in disorganized thinking. Missing one dose of the antipsychotic will most likely not cause a relapse. Daytime somnolence is an adverse reaction to taking the drug. Aggressive behavior is an acute breakthrough of the clinical manifestations. Suicidal thoughts would not result from one missed dose of an antipsychotic.
NP = As
CN = Ph/6
CL = An
SA = 5

21. 4. Talking to the client in a louder tone of voice, distracting the client with a unit activity, or asking another nurse to talk to the client will all serve to increase the amount of environment stimulation, which can make communication with the client who is hearing voices even more difficult. The appropriate intervention is to assess the client in a nonstimulating area because it will help decrease any environmental stimulation.
NP = Im
CN = Ps/4
CL = Ap
SA = 2

22. 3. A community nurse should teach specific social skills to a client with disorganized schizophrenia, because social skills provide the client with tangible help in the community and may include self-esteem and grooming interventions. Making extra home visits will foster client dependence on the community nurse. Convincing the client of self-worth must be an internal accomplishment of the client. Pointing out grooming deficits to the client does not address the root issue of how to become reintegrated.
NP = Im
CN = Ps/4
CL = Ap
SA = 2

23. 3. Evidence of a client with residual schizophrenia who lacks motivation to complete self-directed activities is an inability to complete adequate hygiene. Dressing in mismatched clothing or having a cold breakfast represent daily activities performed by the client. Exhibiting a sense of tiredness on awakening does not ensure decreased motivation.
NP = Ev
CN = Ps/4
CL = An
SA = 2

24. 1. Telling a client who reports seeing Saddam Hussein on the unit that "I know you believe that but he's not here" provides reality orientation. Telling a client that "You are hallucinating again," that it is ridiculous to see Saddam Hussein, or asking where the client saw Saddam are all counterproductive to establishing a therapeutic relationship.
NP = An
CN = Ps/4
CL = An
SA = 2

25. 3. Delirium tremens generally occurs by the third day of withdrawal from alcohol, so it is less likely to be an initial diagnosis of schizophrenia.
NP = An
CN = Ps/4
CL = An
SA = 2

26. 3. Monitoring a client, assessing a client, and developing a plan of care are all assignments that would appropriately only be delegated to a registered nurse. A licensed practical nurse may administer an antipsychotic drug to a client.
NP = Pl
CN = Sa/1
CL = An
SA = 8

PARANOID DISORDERS - COMPREHENSIVE EXAM

1. A client who is diagnosed with paranoid personality disorder is distrustful of the community mental health center staff. The nurse can facilitate trust by
   1. joking around with the client.
   2. being animated when approaching the client.
   3. providing reality testing with the client.
   4. introducing the client to another nurse.

2. A client who has been diagnosed with paranoia due to depression is rambling on about religious delusions. Which of the following is the most appropriate response to the client by the nurse?
   1. "Would you like to talk about something else?"
   2. "Would you like to speak to the chaplain?"
   3. "Would you like a bible to read?"
   4. "Would you like for me to point out your delusions?"

3. A recently admitted client who has paranoid delusions believes that the Federal Bureau of Investigation (FBI) is stalking. The nurse reports to the physician that the client is experiencing what specific type of delusion?

   _____

4. The nurse documents which of the following client statements as an example of a persecutory delusion?
   1. "I think my body is full of cancer."
   2. "I was King Louis XIV in a former life."
   3. "The Federal Bureau of Investigation (FBI) and the Central Intelligence Agency (CIA) are plotting against me."
   4. "The President is secretly in love with me."

5. The nurse should monitor a client suspected of having paranoid schizophrenia for which of the following clinical manifestations?
   Select all that apply:
   [ ] 1. Hallucinations
   [ ] 2. Disorganized speech
   [ ] 3. Inappropriate affect
   [ ] 4. Delusions
   [ ] 5. Disorganized behavior
   [ ] 6. Catatonia

6. A client who had a frustrating day came home and kicked the dog. The nurse documents this as what type of defense mechanism?

   1. Reaction formation

   2. Denial

   3. Projection

   4. Sublimation

7. The client who is bothered with paranoid delusions is resistant to talking about the content of those thoughts. The nurse evaluates that the client is experiencing which of the following primary emotions?

   1. Sadness

   2. Anxiety

   3. Empathy

   4. Peacefulness

ANSWERS AND RATIONALES

1. **3.** A client with a diagnosis of paranoid personality disorder who is distrustful of the staff can facilitate trust by providing reality testing with the client. Joking with the client, being animated when approaching the client, or introducing the client to another nurse may all be interpreted as insincere attempts on the nurse's part to establish a trusting working relationship. Providing reality testing offers a starting point for the nurse to facilitate trust through helping the client to establish reality.
   NP = Im
   CN = Ps/4
   CL = Ap
   SA = 2

2. **1.** For a client who is diagnosed with paranoia from depression and is rambling on about religious delusions, the most appropriate response by the nurse would be to ask if the client would like to talk about something else. Asking if the client would like to speak to the chaplain or read the bible focuses on the delusional content. Asking if the client would like to talk about something else assists the client to focus on a more productive conversation that doesn't further establish the delusions. It would not be appropriate to ask if the client would like the nurse to point out delusional behavior.
   NP = An
   CN = Ps/4
   CL = An
   SA = 2

3. **Persecutory.** The individual who has persecutory delusions believes that he or she is being singled out for harm by others, such as being stalked by the FBI. Persecutory delusions are common in paranoid disorders.
NP = An
CN = Ps/4
CL = Ap
SA = 2

4. 3. People who have persecutory delusions think someone is plotting against them. A client who feels riddled with cancer is experiencing a somatic delusion. A client who verbalizes being King Louis XIV is having a grandiose delusion. A client who verbalizes about being the recipient of the president's love is exhibiting an erotomanic delusion.
NP = Im
CN = Ps/4
CL = Ap
SA = 2

5. 1, 4. Clinical manifestations of paranoid schizophrenia include delusions and hallucinations. Disorganized speech, inappropriate affect, disorganized behavior, and catatonia are not features of paranoid schizophrenia.
NP = As
CN = Ps/4
CL = Ap
SA = 2

6. 3. Projection is the attribution of unconscious feelings, uncomfortable wishes, or motivation to another individual. Reaction formation is the process of banning unacceptable feelings or behaviors from consciousness by displaying the opposite behavior. Denial is the process of banning unacceptable thoughts by refusing to accept their presence. Sublimation is the unconscious process of replacing unconstructive or socially unacceptable behaviors with behaviors that are more acceptable than in their original form. Clients with paranoia project their own issues onto others and become suspicious of others for what the client believes is another person's issue.
NP = Im
CN = Ps/4
CL = Ap
SA = 2

7. 2. Because of anxiety, clients who experience paranoid delusions are always on guard, expecting to be harassed or injured.
NP = Ev
CN = Ps/4
CL = An
SA = 2

Practice Test 3

1. Which of the following should the nurse include in the plan of care for a client diagnosed with paranoia?
    1. Talk to the client in a low voice
    2. Stay within the client's social space
    3. Use indirect eye contact
    4. Touch the client after asking permission

2. Which of the following is the priority approach for the nurse to implement for a client who is diagnosed with paranoid delusions and is feeling socially isolated?
    1. Tell the client to get involved in a solitary activity
    2. Identify the precipitating factor to the delusions
    3. Teach the client new calming techniques
    4. Work with the client on communication strategies

3. The nurse is caring for a client who is experiencing persecutory delusions related to a paranoid disorder and who believes that there is a need for self-protection. Which of the following nursing diagnoses is the priority for this client?
    1. Risk for other-directed violence
    2. Adjustment, impaired
    3. Social isolation
    4. Anxiety

4. The nurse includes which of the following when teaching social interaction skills to a client with the diagnosis of paranoia?

1. Getting exercise

2. Taking a prescribed drug

3. Going to individual therapy

4. Active listening

5. The nurse evaluates a client diagnosed with paranoid personality disorder as most likely demonstrating which of the following while involved in an interpersonal relationship?

   1. Avoidance

   2. Takes the blame for personal mistakes

   3. Equally shared communication

   4. Trusts the fidelity of a partner

6. The nurse is teaching a class on paranoid schizophrenia. The nurse should include what two hallmark characteristics? _____

7. A 20-year-old male client is admitted to an inpatient unit with a first-time onset of paranoid thoughts. The nurse identifies that this client has paranoid personality disorder because

   1. it is more common in men.

   2. there is no environmental stressor.

   3. the onset of clinical manifestations is earlier in life.

   4. the client has a genetic predisposition.

8. A concerned party makes contact with an admissions nurse to initiate treatment for a client who is experiencing paranoid delusions. The nurse expects to see the client enter the system by which of the following routes?

   1. Bringing oneself to the emergency department

   2. A concerned family member

   3. Finding a therapist for oneself

   4. Getting help via an employee assistance program

9. The nurse anticipates that clients with paranoid delusional disorder are likely to get involved in the legal system because they _____.

10. A client diagnosed with paranoid delusional disorder believes that the food has been poisoned. What is the most appropriate nursing diagnosis for this client? _____

11. A client with paranoid delusional disorder tells the nurse that his wife is having an affair with the hospital administrator and that is why the client hasn't been discharged yet. Which of the following would be the most appropriate nursing intervention for the client?

1. Convince the client that you believe him in order to establish rapport
2. Inform the client that his thoughts are mistaken beliefs
3. Be available to the client in order to assist him in reducing anxiety
4. Avoid the client until he approaches you to tell you the truth

12. A client who has paranoid delusions has been attending a social skills group. The nurse will expect which of the following initial outcomes for this client? The client will

   1. identify anxiety-producing public situations.
   2. become chair of the social committee.
   3. warn the group members about potentially violent behavior.
   4. file for a divorce because of an alleged affair.

13. A client with paranoid delusional disorder is learning about the prescribed antipsychotic drug. The nurse provides drug teaching by including instructions for the client to take the antipsychotic drug

   1. when the client is feeling anxious.
   2. as scheduled by the physician.
   3. until the client learns new coping methods.
   4. at bedtime to help bring on sleep.

14. The nurse is caring for a client who is experiencing paranoid psychosis and has a history of substance abuse. Based on the understanding of mental effects of substance use, the nurse recognizes that the client has most likely ingested large amounts of

   1. vitamins.
   2. nicotine.
   3. alcohol.
   4. marijuana.

15. A client who is experiencing paranoid psychosis is afraid to take prescribed drugs because of a belief that they are poisoned. Which of the following interventions is the most effective to encourage this client to take the drugs?

   1. Explain the purpose of the drugs
   2. Bring the pill to the client in a cup
   3. Let the client watch the nurse open the drugs
   4. Have the client watch the other clients take their drugs

16. Which of the following nursing interventions is most appropriate for a client experiencing paranoid psychosis who feels threatened and unable to fall asleep?

1. Have the client go to bed earlier

2. Allow the client to choose a location for falling asleep

3. Suggest that the client exercise before bedtime

4. Encourage the client to stick to a routine

17. The nurse is assessing a client who is withdrawing from an unknown substance. Because the client is experiencing extreme paranoia, the nurse should assess the client for traces of which substance in the urinalysis drug screen?

1. Tobacco

2. Pain medication

3. Amphetamines

4. Sedatives

18. The nurse should monitor a client experiencing alcohol withdrawal for which of the following adverse reactions?
Select all that apply:

[ ] 1. Decreased sleep

[ ] 2. Increased appetite

[ ] 3. Bradycardia

[ ] 4. Visual hallucinations

[ ] 5. Hypotension

[ ] 6. Delusions

19. The registered nurse is preparing to make the clinical assignments on a psychiatric unit. Which of the following assignments should the nurse appropriately delegate to a licensed practical nurse?

1. Perform a urinalysis drug screen on a client with paranoid delusions

2. Assess a client with paranoia for alcohol withdrawal

3. Remove all personnel belongings of the client on admission that may be perceived as harmful

4. Develop a discharge plan for a client with paranoid schizophrenia

ANSWERS AND RATIONALES

1. 4. It is appropriate to touch a client experiencing paranoia only after asking the permission of the client. Whispering, staying close to the client, or using indirect eye contact may make the client become more suspicious.
NP = Pl
CN = Ps/4
CL = Ap
SA = 2

2. 4. Because a client with paranoid delusions is feeling socially isolated, the nurse should work with the client on communication strategies. Engaging a client in a solitary activity would keep the client socially isolated. Although identifying precipitating factors and teaching the client calming techniques may be helpful, they do not deal directly with the social isolation issue and are not the priority.
   NP = Im
   CN = Sa/1
   CL = An
   SA = 8

3. 1. Clients who have a paranoid disorder and experience persecutory delusions may feel defensive and the need to protect themselves. Risk for violence would be the priority diagnosis.
   NP = An
   CN = Sa/1
   CL = An
   SA = 2

4. 4. The nurse should use active listening when teaching social interaction skills to a client with a diagnosis of paranoia.
   NP = Im
   CN = Ps/4
   CL = Ap
   SA = 2

5. 1. A client with paranoid personality disorder would most likely demonstrate an avoidance of interpersonal relationships. Because of the suspicions, this client would have difficulties with personal relationships.
   NP = Ev
   CN = Ps/4
   CL = Ap
   SA = 2

6. **Persecutory delusions and auditory hallucinations.** The two classic features of paranoid schizophrenia include persecutory delusions and auditory hallucinations.
   NP = Pl
   CN = Ps/4
   CL = Ap
   SA = 2

7. 3. The onset of paranoid personality disorder occurs earlier in a client's life, generally during adolescence or young adulthood. It is more common in women, is influenced by environmental stressors, and does not have a genetic component.

NP = An
CN = Ps/4
CL = An
SA = 2

8. **2.** A client who has paranoid delusions does not generally recognize the difficulties that the delusions cause for the client or significant others.
NP = An
CN = Ps/4
CL = An
SA = 2

9. **are convinced that others intentionally want to harm them.** Clients with paranoid delusional disorder take others to court due to their defensive retaliation against what they believe is harassment or persecution.
NP = An
CN = Ps/4
CL = An
SA = 2

10. **Disturbed thought processes.** A client with paranoid delusional disorder may feel the food is poisoned as a direct result of paranoid thoughts. The appropriate nursing diagnosis is Disturbed thought processes.
NP = An
CN = Ps/4
CL = An
SA = 2

11. **3.** The most appropriate nursing intervention for a client with paranoid delusional disorder who tells the nurse that his wife is having an affair with the hospital administrator is to be available to the client in order to reduce anxiety. This will allow the client to know of the nurse's noninvasive support. Convincing the client that the nurse believes the claim simply to build rapport and avoiding the client until the client approaches the nurse are both countertherapeutic. Telling the client that the thoughts are mistaken beliefs will not support a trusting relationship.
NP = Pl
CN = Ps/4
CL = Ap
SA = 2

12. **2.** The best outcome for a client who has paranoid delusions and who has been attending a social skills group is to become chair of the social committee. Identifying anxiety-producing public situations and filing for divorce because of a spouse's alleged affair are not the expected initial

results of a social skills group. They may be expectations later in therapy. Warning the group about the client's potentially violent behavior would serve to further socially isolate the client.

NP = Ev
CN = Ps/4
CL = An
SA = 2

13. **2.** The nurse should instruct a client with paranoid delusional disorder to take the antipsychotic drugs as scheduled by the physician. A client must understand that part of treatment is to take the drugs as scheduled and that the treatment plan can be adjusted in conjunction with health care providers.

NP = Pl
CN = Ph/6
CL = Ap
SA = 5

14. **3.** Paranoid psychosis can be caused by ingestion of large amounts of alcohol.

NP = An
CN = Ps/4
CL = An
SA = 2

15. **3.** The most appropriate intervention for a client who is experiencing paranoid psychosis and afraid to take prescribed drugs would be to let the client watch the nurse open the drugs. This allows the client to identify the drugs and alleviate the paranoia. Explaining the purpose of the drugs, bringing the pill to the client in a cup, or having the client watch other clients take their pills does not do anything to dispel the client's paranoia.

NP = Pl
CN = Ph/6
CL = Ap
SA = 5

16. **2.** The most appropriate intervention for a client experiencing paranoid psychosis who feels threatened and is unable to fall asleep is to allow the client to choose a location for falling asleep. This allows the client to be in control and feel safer. Suggesting that the client go to bed an hour earlier, exercise before bedtime, or stick to a routine doesn't address the phenomenon that the client is feeling threatened at bedtime.

NP = Pl
CN = Ps/4
CL = Ap
SA = 2

17. 3. Clients who are in amphetamine withdrawal are known to experience paranoia.
    NP = As
    CN = Ps/4
    CL = Ap
    SA = 2

18. 1, 4, 6. Adverse reactions to alcohol withdrawal include decreased sleep, decreased appetite, tachycardia, visual hallucinations, hypertension, and delusions.
    NP = As
    CN = Ps/4
    CL = Ap
    SA = 2

19. 3. Assignments such as performing a urinalysis drug screen, assessing a client, and developing a discharge plan require the skills of the registered nurse. A licensed practical nurse may remove all belongings of a client that are perceived to be harmful after an admission has been performed by the registered nurse.
    NP = Pl
    CN = Sa/1
    CL = An
    SA = 8

POST-TRAUMATIC STRESS DISORDERS - COMPREHENSIVE EXAM

1. Which of the following should be the priority nursing action for the nurse in the emergency room caring for a client who reports having been raped and appears restless, confused, and tearful?

    1. Call security and report the rape

    2. Stay with the client to begin establishing a trusting relationship

    3. Leave the client to calm down and return later

    4. Begin the physical assessment

2. A client reports a marked increase in nightmares, irritability, and feelings of despair. Upon further assessment, the client reveals having been a soldier during the Vietnam War and now has a child who has decided to join the service. The nurse assesses this client to be experiencing what?

    _____

3. Based on an understanding of the care provided to a client who has been raped, the nurse should document which of the following?

1. The client's information paraphrased
2. The client's information word for word
3. All pertinent information except the client's emotional behavior
4. Only the information the client agrees to have documented

4. When working with a client with a diagnosis of rape trauma syndrome, the nurse recognizes the clinical manifestations of rape trauma syndrome most closely resemble what disorder? _____

5. A client comes into the emergency room with facial bruising and tearfully tells the nurse about being raped. The client states, "I wish I would have just died." The most appropriate response by the nurse is
   1. "You're lucky to be alive."
   2. "It will get better over time."
   3. "It must have been scary, tell me what you mean?"
   4. "You don't mean that, because death is permanent."

6. A client who has been raped is experiencing irritability, mood swings, and insomnia. The most appropriate nursing diagnosis for this client would be
   1. Coping, ineffective.
   2. Self-esteem, situational low.
   3. Powerlessness.
   4. Rape-trauma syndrome.

7. The spouse of a client being evaluated after having been raped tells the nurse "I just can't handle this anymore." The appropriate response by the nurse is
   1. "This must be very difficult for you."
   2. "Why do you feel you can't handle this?"
   3. "Would you rather talk later?"
   4. "Your spouse needs you to be strong."

8. The client who was raped tells the nurse, "I should have done something, but I was too afraid to fight." Which of the following is the priority response by the nurse?
   1. "It is better to fight back."
   2. "There is nothing you could have done."
   3. "You weren't thinking clearly at the time."
   4. "By doing what you did, you survived and that's most important."

9. Which of the following does the nurse evaluate as a long-term goal for a client who has been raped?

1. Prosecute the attacker in a court of law
2. Accept responsibility in the rape
3. Accept and begin to resolve feelings about the rape
4. Try to forget the rape

10. A nurse asks another nurse what the outcome is for a client who has received counseling after being raped? The nurse's response would be

    1. "A rape survivor often becomes depressed and suicidal."
    2. "A rape survivor develops clinical manifestations associated with post-traumatic stress disorder."
    3. "A rape survivor is often unable to engage in intimate relationships."
    4. "A rape survivor is able to return to one's previous level of functioning."

11. After changing into an exam gown, the client who has been raped hands the nurse the removed clothes. Which of the following is the appropriate nursing action?

    1. Allow the client to throw the clothes away as part of the healing process
    2. Put the clothes in a bag and send them home with the client
    3. Give them to hospital security
    4. Place the clothes in an appropriate storage bag and save them

12. A client has been raped and tearfully tells the nurse, "I don't know what to do, I just can't decide." The nurse should include which of the following in the plan of care for this client?

    1. Encourage the client's significant other to make the decisions
    2. Make decisions for the client with the client's best interests in mind
    3. Encourage the client to participate in making decisions about care
    4. Give the client step-by-step instructions of what is taking place

13. The nurse is talking with a client who has been raped and is assessing the client's need for emergency contraception. The client states, "My period ended just a few days ago and I don't believe in contraception." Which of the following is the appropriate response by the nurse?

    1. Tell the client that she is not at risk for getting pregnant
    2. Explain the potential risks and benefits of taking emergency contraception
    3. Encourage the client to take the emergency contraception immediately
    4. Avoid discussion of emergency contraception because it's contrary to the client's belief system

14. A client has been brought to the emergency room by friends. The client and friends are all laughing and acting silly. They tell the nurse that the client has been raped. Before responding to this client, which of the following should the nurse consider?

    1. Assume nothing really serious happened because the client and friends are laughing

    2. Consider that the client and friends have been drinking and would not be good historians

    3. The client may be more serious if taken to a private location

    4. Realize there is a wide range of emotions that people can experience after being raped

15. Which of the following clinical manifestations of post-traumatic stress disorder should the nurse assess a client for?
    Select all that apply:

    [ ] 1. Increased interest in usual activities

    [ ] 2. Increased sleep

    [ ] 3. Difficulty concentrating

    [ ] 4. Distressing dreams

    [ ] 5. Sense of short feelings

    [ ] 6. More time spent with people

16. The registered nurse is preparing to delegate nursing tasks to a licensed practical nurse. Which of the following tasks would the nurse appropriately delegate?

    1. Evaluate a client for possible post-traumatic stress disorder

    2. Offer support to a client who was raped

    3. Instruct a client who was raped to attempt to put that in the past

    4. Develop a plan of care for a client with post-traumatic stress disorder

ANSWERS AND RATIONALES

1. 2. The priority response for any client having experienced a traumatic event is to provide support and to begin to establish a trusting relationship. The client's emotional needs should be met before the physical assessment begins. Although security must be contacted, it is not the priority. The client who was raped and is distraught should not be left alone.
   NP = Pl
   CN = Sa/1
   CL = Ap
   SA = 8

2. **Post-traumatic stress disorder.** Clinical manifestations of post-traumatic stress disorder may develop months or years after a traumatic event. The response may be triggered by an event that is similar to the original trauma, such as having a child join the service.
NP = As
CN = Ps/4
CL = Ap
SA = 2

3. 2. All verbal information gathered by the nurse should be documented exactly how the client stated it.
NP = Im
CN = Ps/4
CL = An
SA = 2

4. **Post-traumatic stress disorder.** Rape trauma syndrome is a variation of post-traumatic stress disorder. If left untreated, a client may develop depression, anxiety, and sexual dysfunction.
NP = An
CN = Ps/4
CL = Ap
SA = 2

5. 3. Clients who have been raped may become suicidal. The nurse's priority is to assess the client for suicidal ideation. Saying that it will get better over time, that death is permanent, or that the client is lucky to be alive all dismiss the client's feelings.
NP = An
CN = Ps/4
CL = An
SA = 2

6. 4. The nursing diagnosis of Rape-trauma syndrome encompasses and acknowledges the wide range of clinical manifestations that rape survivors experience.
NP = An
CN = Ps/4
CL = An
SA = 2

7. 1. The spouse of a rape survivor also experiences the impact and assault of the rape on the relationship and needs support. "Why" questions put the client on the defensive and should be avoided. Asking if the spouse would rather talk later does not address why the spouse is upset. Telling the spouse to be strong dismisses the spouse's feelings.

NP = An
CN = Ps/4
CL = An
SA = 2

8. 4. The priority response for a client who was raped is to assure the client that the client did the right thing and survived. The client needs to feel empowered and that the best was done in a bad situation.
NP = An
CN = Sa/1
CL = An
SA = 2

9. 3. There are many potential long-term effects of having been raped. By accepting and dealing with the rape, it is hoped that the client will begin the healing process. Taking legal action is not mandatory in resolving the feelings about the rape. The rape survivor is not responsible for the rape, and telling the client to forget about it and focus on other things will not resolve the client's feelings.
NP = Ev
CN = Ps/4
CL = An
SA = 2

10. 4. With supportive services, counseling, and crisis intervention, most rape survivors will return to their previous level of functioning. However, there is always the risk that the client will become depressed, have difficulty with intimate relationships, or develop post-traumatic stress disorder.
NP = Ev
CN = Ps/4
CL = An
SA = 2

11. 4. Initially after the rape and the client's putting on an exam gown, the nurse should place the client's clothes in an appropriate storage bag and save them. Preserving the DNA evidence that may be on the client's clothes increases the chances of identifying the perpetrator if the client decides to press charges.
NP = Pl
CN = Ps/4
CL = Ap
SA = 2

12. 3. Encouraging and supporting the client to make decisions about the care allows the client to begin to regain control during a very out-of-control time.

NP = Pl
CN = Ps/4
CL = Ap
SA = 2

13. 2. The client is at risk for getting pregnant after being raped. Explaining the risks and benefits of emergency contraception allows the client to make an informed decision. A discussion of emergency contraception should not be avoided because of either the client's or the nurse's belief system.
NP = An
CN = Ps/4
CL = An
SA = 2

14. 4. In the acute stage of rape, which occurs immediately following the rape, the client may experience a wide range of emotions, including laughing, crying, and withdrawal. Clients who report having been raped should always be taken seriously and be offered emotional support and physical evaluation.
NP = An
CN = Ps/4
CL = An
SA = 2

15. 3, 4, 5. Clinical manifestations of post-traumatic stress disorder include decreased interest in usual activities, sleeplessness, difficulty concentrating, distressing dreams, sense of shortfeelings, and avoidance of people.
NP = As
CN = Ps/4
CL = Ap
SA = 2

16. 2. It would be appropriate to delegate offering the support to a rape client of all team members, including a licensed practical nurse. Evaluating a client for post-traumatic stress disorder and developing a plan of care are tasks that should be performed by a registered nurse. No team member should ever instruct a client who was raped to put it in the past. The client must be allowed to effectively deal with the rape.
NP = Pl
CN = Sa/1
CL = An
SA = 8

SUBSTANCE ABUSE - COMPREHENSIVE EXAM

1. The nurse is educating a client recently admitted to the chemical dependency unit for alcohol dependence about the medical complications that can result due to long-term use of alcohol. Which of the following medical complications should the nurse include in the teaching?

    1. Migrainelike headaches and ulceration of the nasal mucosa
    2. Fatty liver and liver cirrhosis
    3. Yawning and muscle cramping
    4. Unpleasant dreams, perceptual changes with vivid colors, visions of halos

2. A client arrives at an outpatient clinic complaining of rhinorrhea, chills, lacrimation, muscle cramps, and yawning. The nurse evaluates the client to be experiencing

    1. opiate withdrawal.
    2. cannabis intoxication.
    3. hallucinogen abuse.
    4. nicotine withdrawal.

3. The nurse admitted a client experiencing cannabis intoxication to the chemical dependency unit. Which of the following nursing interventions would be the priority for the nurse when planning the care for this client?

    1. Provide adequate nutrition and hydration
    2. Encourage rest
    3. Encourage use of deep breathing and guided imagery
    4. Protect the client from falling

4. A client presents to the chemical dependency unit with a pulse of 110, blood pressure of 186/108, hand tremors, and diaphoresis. The nurse suspects which of the following?

    1. Alcohol withdrawal
    2. Cocaine withdrawal
    3. Cannabis withdrawal
    4. Nicotine withdrawal

5. A client is experiencing labile emotions and expresses concern over nervousness, sleep disturbances, and cravings for nicotine. The priority intervention for this client is to

    1. teach sleep hygiene techniques.
    2. obtain an order for bupropion (Zyban).

3. assist the client in identifying triggers to nicotine use.

4. teach relaxation techniques, such as deep breathing or guided imagery.

6. The nurse should include which of the following in the treatment plan when caring for a client with opioid intoxication?

1. Provision for safety

2. Education on the benefits of abstinence from opioids

3. Promotion of exercise

4. Adherence to a diet low in sodium

7. Which of the following subjective clinical manifestations does the nurse evaluate as a clinical manifestation of a client experiencing alcohol withdrawal?

1. Hand tremors

2. Feelings of restlessness

3. Elevated blood pressure

4. Diaphoresis

8. A client is brought to the emergency room experiencing clinical manifestations of left upper quadrant abdominal pain radiating to the back that is associated with nausea and vomiting. The client admits to drinking 125 ml of whiskey every other day for the past 3 months. The nurse suspects the medical complication of _____.

9. The nurse is caring for a client experiencing an opioid withdrawal. Which of the following measures should receive priority in the client's plan of care?
Select all that apply:

[   ] 1. Administer a narcotic

[   ] 2. Provide a high-calorie diet

[   ] 3. Increase fluid intake

[   ] 4. Provide warm blankets

[   ] 5. Encourage the use of a whirlpool

[   ] 6. Administer clonidine (Catapres)

10. A client admitted to the intensive care unit vomiting bright red blood has a long-standing history of alcohol abuse. The nurse suspects which of the following medical complications due to alcohol abuse?

1. Ascites

2. Liver cirrhosis

3. Portal hypertension

4. Esophageal varices

11. The nurse assesses a client who is hospitalized for alcohol withdrawal. The client complains of abdominal pain and the nurse observes that the client's abdomen is profusely distended. The nurse suspects that the client is most likely experiencing what condition? _____

12. The nurse should monitor a client with a history of meperidine (Demerol) abuse for which of the following withdrawal manifestations?
Select all that apply:

[ ] 1. Weight gain

[ ] 2. Bradycardia

[ ] 3. Lacrimation

[ ] 4. Rhinorrhea

[ ] 5. Constipation

[ ] 6. Muscle cramps

13. Which of the following is a priority for the nurse to include in the discharge instructions given to a client who is chemically dependent on opioids?

1. Discuss ways to decrease spending time around opioid-using friends

2. Explore attitudes and behaviors that may precipitate a relapse

3. Encourage abstinence from all pain medications, including nonsteroidal anti-inflammatories

4. Provide information about the process of opioid withdrawal.

14. The mother of a client who has been admitted to the hospital for excessive use of cocaine asks the nurse what the complications are of cocaine use. The appropriate response by the nurse is, "Cocaine abuse can cause various medical complications including
Select all that apply:

[ ] 1. Wernicke-Korsokoff's syndrome."

[ ] 2. migrainelike headaches."

[ ] 3. weight gain."

[ ] 4. abnormal heart rhythms."

[ ] 5. slowed thought processes"

[ ] 6. respiratory depression."

15. A client presents to the clinic experiencing analgesia, itching, drooling, and nodding. The nurse reports that the client is suspected of abusing which of the following substances?

1. Benzodiazepines

2. Opioids

3. Alcohol

4. Barbiturates

16. The nurse is caring for a client who is experiencing marked confusion, unsteady gait, and diplopia after being admitted to the hospital for alcohol withdrawal. Which of the following nursing interventions is the priority for the nurse to implement?

    1. Encourage adequate nutrition and fluids
    2. Administer prescribed thiamine
    3. Provide safety measures
    4. Administer prescribed benzodiazepine

17. The nurse receives a report on a client who is being admitted from the emergency room and has been abusing benzodiazepines for an extended period of time. Based on this information, it would be most important for the nurse to

    1. administer the same benzodiazepine that the client has abused for detoxification.
    2. administer an opioid analgesic and encourage rest.
    3. provide adequate food and fluid intake.
    4. begin instruction on the consequences of chemical dependence on family relationships.

18. The nurse is caring for a client who is going through benzodiazepine withdrawal. Which of the following is the priority for the nurse to perform?

    1. Provide a warm tub bath
    2. Assess vital signs and prevent seizure activity
    3. Place client in a side-lying position to prevent aspiration
    4. Offer fluids to prevent dehydration

19. The nurse is caring for a client admitted with alcoholism and cardiac arrhythmias. The client states, "I have been under a lot of stress lately and have been trying to lose a few pounds, so I have not been eating and have been drinking only coffee, cola, and three to four alcoholic drinks a day." Which of the following would be a priority in this client's plan of care?

    1. Inform the client that alcohol provides empty calories and encourage a well-balanced diet
    2. Encourage verbalization of feelings, including causes of stress, and offer stress management techniques
    3. Inform the client that the combination of alcohol and caffeinated beverages cause arrhythmias
    4. Instruct the client to avoid activity and report any chest pain and dyspnea

20. The charge nurse is reviewing the chart of a client admitted for opioid withdrawal. Which of the following drug orders should the nurse clarify?

    1. Clonidine (Catapres) 1.2 mg PO daily

    2. Naproxen 500 mg PO twice a day p.r.n.

    3. Diphenoxylate/atropine (Lomotil) 2.5 mg PO four times a day

    4. Oxycodone/acetaminophen (Tylox) 5 mg/325 mg PO every 4 hours p.r.n.

21. The nurse instructs a client that which of the following are clinical manifestations of caffeine intoxication?Select all that apply:

    [   ] 1. Bradycardia

    [   ] 2. Flushed face

    [   ] 3. Muscle twitching

    [   ] 4. Somnolence

    [   ] 5. Hypoglycemia

    [   ] 6. Increased bowel motility

22. Which of the following questions would provide the nurse with the most accurate information on a client's insight into alcoholism?

    1. "Have you experienced an upset stomach and had trouble eating?"

    2. "Have you ever taken a drink the first thing in the morning?"

    3. "Have you been feeling anxious and had trouble sleeping?"

    4. "Have you felt ill lately and missed a lot of work?"

23. The nurse is preparing discharge instructions for a client who experienced a myocardial infarction and has a history of smoking two packs of cigarettes per day. Which of the following should the nurse include in the smoking-cessation instructions?

    1. Heavy smoking causes physiological changes, such as an increased appetite and subsequent weight gain

    2. Smoking is psychologically addicting and all withdrawal clinical manifestations are psychologically based

    3. Substitute a nonalcoholic beverage for a cigarette when in situations previously associated with smoking

    4. Withdrawal clinical manifestations commonly occur with a brief abstinence in smoking

24. The most significant role for a nurse in nicotine use and abuse includes which of the following?Select all that apply:

    [   ] 1. Teach smoking-cessation programs

    [   ] 2. Serve as an advocate for nonsmoking legislation

[   ] 3. Encourage antidepressant medication

[   ] 4. Provide antismoking education to schools

[   ] 5. Instruct the client on relapse prevention techniques

[   ] 6. Provide unbiased care to clients with diseases caused by smoking

25. The nurse is assessing the client for toxic levels of amphetamines. Toxic levels of amphetamines would most likely be represented by which of the following clinical manifestations?
Select all that apply:

[   ] 1. Depression

[   ] 2. Hypertension

[   ] 3. Overly suspicious and paranoid behavior

[   ] 4. Psychomotor retardation

[   ] 5. Touching and picking of the extremities and face

[   ] 6. Unpleasant and vivid dreams

26. The registered nurse is preparing to delegate nursing assignments for a psychiatric unit. Which of the following nursing assignments is an appropriate delegation?

1. Unlicensed assistive personnel assist a client in alcoholic withdrawal to group therapy

2. A licensed practical nurse instructs a client with nicotine dependence on smoking-cessation techniques

3. Unlicensed assistive personnel encourage a client admitted with an opiate dependency to verbalize feelings

4. A licensed practical nurse assesses a client with a morphine dependency for withdrawal clinical manifestations

ANSWERS AND RATIONALES

1. 2. The liver is the organ that detoxifies alcohol. The client who abuses alcohol over a long period of time will develop a fatty liver, which will progress to alcoholic hepatitis. The end result is liver cirrhosis. Clinical manifestations of yawning and muscle cramping are associated with opiate withdrawal. Clinical manifestations of perceptual changes and unpleasant dreams are associated with hallucinogen intoxication. Migrainelike headaches and ulceration of the nasal mucosa are caused by cocaine abuse.
NP = Pl
CN = Ps/4
CL = An
SA = 2

2. 1. The clinical manifestations of rhinorrhea, chills, lacrimation, muscle cramps, and yawning are all indicative of opiate withdrawal.
NP = Ev
CN = Ps/4
CL = An
SA = 2

3. 4. While it is important to provide adequate nutrition and hydration, rest, deep breathing, and guided imagery, protecting the client from falling is a priority nursing intervention when caring for the client experiencing cannabis intoxication.
NP = Pl
CN = Sa/1
CL = An
SA = 8

4. 1. An elevated pulse and blood pressure, along with hand tremors and diaphoresis, are all indicative of alcohol withdrawal.
NP = Ev
CN = Ps/4
CL = An
SA = 2

5. 2. While the interventions of teaching sleep hygiene techniques, assisting the client in identifying triggers to nicotine use, and teaching relaxation techniques are beneficial nursing interventions for the client in nicotine withdrawal, obtaining an order for a nicotine patch system or bupropion (Zyban) would be a priority. It reduces the withdrawal manifestations and would assist the client in being more comfortable, thus increasing the client's ability to learn new coping strategies.
NP = Pl
CN = Sa/1
CL = An
SA = 8

6. 1. A client experiencing opioid intoxication has the clinical manifestations of euphoria, itching, respiratory depression, and drowsiness, therefore preventing effective teaching from taking place. Exercise would not be encouraged because it will not assist in the rapid detoxification from opioids. A low-sodium diet does not assist the client who is intoxicated from opioids. Safety, including the prevention of falls, is a priority nursing intervention for the client who is intoxicated from opioids.
NP = Pl
CN = Ps/4
CL = Ap
SA = 2

7. 2. Hand tremors, elevated blood pressure, and diaphoresis are all objective clinical manifestations of alcohol withdrawal. A feeling of restlessness is a subjective clinical manifestation.
NP = Ev
CN = Ps/4
CL = Ap
SA = 2

8. pancreatitis. Left upper quadrant abdominal pain, nausea, and vomiting are the classic clinical manifestations indicating pancreatitis, which may be associated with alcohol intake.
NP = An
CN = Ps/4
CL = Ap
SA = 2

9. 4, ,5 6. It is not appropriate to administer a narcotic to a client in opioid (narcotic) withdrawal. Clonidine (Catapres) is a more appropriate agent to administer in the detoxification from opioids, because it blocks the receptor sites more adequately than does a narcotic. Since the client in opioid withdrawal will be experiencing muscle aches and cramping, encouraging increased activity would not be advised. Providing a high-calorie diet would not be a priority, because the client will be very uncomfortable due to experiencing muscle cramping and chills and is focused on pain relief and feeling better. Providing warm blankets and encouraging the use of a whirlpool will assist in alleviating chills and muscle cramps in the client experiencing opiate withdrawal.
NP = Pl
CN = Sa/1
CL = Ap
SA = 8

10. 4. Ascites is the accumulation of fluid in the abdominal cavity. Portal hypertension occurs as blood is blocked in the liver and cannot flow freely through it due to either a fatty liver or liver cirrhosis. Esophageal varices are pockets of blood that accumulate in the varicose veins in the esophagus and can erupt when the client coughs.
NP = An
CN = Ps/4
CL = Ap
SA = 2

11. Ascites. The alcoholic client who has a profusely distended abdomen and complains of abdominal pain is most likely experiencing ascites, a fluid accumulation in the abdominal cavity.

NP = An
CN = Ps/4
CL = Ap
SA = 2

12. 3, 4, 6. Meperidine (Demerol) is an opioid. Adverse reactions to opioid withdrawal include weight loss, tachycardia, diarrhea, lacrimation, rhinorrhea, and muscles cramps.
NP = As
CN = Ps/4
CL = Ap
SA = 2

13. 2. The client should not spend time with previous using friends who are not in recovery, because it can precipitate a relapse. The client should not take nonopiate pain medications or opiates. The process of opioid withdrawal and teaching about the process has most likely occurred during hospitalization and would not be a priority nursing intervention upon discharge from the hospital. Because behaviors and clinical manifestations of a potential relapse occur long before the actual relapse, the client needs to be instructed about the attitudes and manifestations that can precipitate a relapse.
NP = Pl
CN = Sa/1
CL = Ap
SA = 8

14. 2, 4, 6. Infections, migrainelike headaches, abnormal heart rhythms, and respiratory depression are all medical complications of cocaine abuse. Wernicke-Korsokoff's syndrome is a medical complication of alcohol abuse. A slowing of thought processes is a clinical manifestation of alcohol intoxication. A client who has a problem with cocaine abuse would not gain weight and may actually lose weight.
NP = An
CN = Ps/4
CL = An
SA = 2

15. 2. Clinical manifestations of analgesia, itching, drooling, and nodding suggest abuse of opioids.
NP = An
CN = Ps/4
CL = An
SA = 2

16. 2. Marked confusion, unsteady gait, and diplopia are all clinical manifestations of Wernicke-Korsakoff's syndrome, which is caused by a thiamine or vitamin B_1 deficiency. Prompt treatment with large amounts of thiamine is necessary within the first few hours of the first few days after onset of clinical manifestations. If thiamine is not given within this time period, death may result or the client will develop severe memory impairment, disorientation to person, place, and time, and short-term memory loss.

NP = Im
CN = Sa/1
CL = Ap
SA = 8

17. 1. A benzodiazepine (generally the same one utilized by the client or another similar benzodiazepine) is used per detoxification protocol. Tapering dosages per protocol is most important in the detoxification process of the client.

NP = Pl
CN = Ps/4
CL = Ap
SA = 2

18. 2. The priority nursing intervention for a client who is going through benzodiazepine withdrawal is to assess vital signs and prevent seizure activity. Taking the vital signs provides information regarding the central nervous system. The prevention of seizures is a priority because seizures may accompany benzodiazepine withdrawal if the withdrawal is not handled correctly by using the appropriate drugs. A warm tub bath would not be recommended for the client in benzodiazepine withdrawal, because it can cause the quickened release of benzodiazepines that have been stored in fat cells. Placing a client in a side-lying position to prevent aspiration and offering fluids to prevent dehydration may be appropriate nursing interventions, but they are not the priority nursing intervention.

NP = Im
CN = Sa/1
CL = Ap
SA = 8

19. 3. It would be appropriate to teach a client who is experiencing stress, not eating, and drinking alcohol to eat a well-balanced diet and verbalize the stress. However, the priority intervention for the client who consumes too much alcohol and is experiencing cardiac arrhythmias is to inform the client that the combination of caffeinated beverages and alcohol causes arrhythmias.

NP = Pl
CN = Sa/1
CL = Ap
SA = 8

20. 4. Clonidine is an alpha-adrenergic agonist used primarily to treat hypertension, but it has gained a considerable place in the treatment of reducing clinical manifestations of withdrawal from opioids. Naproxen is a nonsteroidal anti-inflammatory used to treat mild pain in a client addicted to opiates. Lomotil is used to control diarrhea that may occur in opiate addiction. Tylox contains oxycodone, which is a narcotic anagesic and is contraindicated in a client addicted to opioids; an order for Tylox should be questioned.
NP = An
CN = Ps/4
CL = An
SA = 2

21. 2, 3, 6. Clinical manifestations of caffeine intoxication include tachycardia, flushed face, muscle twitching, nervousness, increased blood sugar, and increased motility.
NP = Im
CN = Ps/4
CL = Ap
SA = 2

22. 2. "Have you ever taken a drink the first thing in the morning?" is a significant question and part of the CAGE questionnaire. The client with alcoholism frequently takes a drink first thing in the morning to steady the nerves. Clients with a diagnosis of alcoholism often lack insight into their illness and the need to change.
NP = Ev
CN = Ps/4
CL = An
SA = 2

23. 4. Smoking decreases appetite. Nicotine is both physically and psychologically addicting. Avoiding situations previously associated with smoking, such as having an alcohol drink or a cup of coffee, offer the best chance of success at smoking cessation. Withdrawal clinical manifestations commonly do occur, even with a brief abstinence such as occurs in nonsmoking workplaces or airplanes.
NP = Pl
CN = Ps/4
CL = Ap
SA = 2

24. 2, 4. The most significant role a nurse can play in nicotine use and abuse is that of education and prevention of nicotine use. Primary prevention would include community-wide education especially targeted at school-age children to prevent smoking from ever starting and serving as an advocate

for antismoking legislation. Teaching smoking-cessation programs, encouraging antidepressant drugs, and instructing the client on relapse prevention techniques are all examples of secondary prevention, encouraging smokers to quit smoking through smoking-cessation programs and related activities. Providing unbiased care to clients who smoke and offering nonjudgmental and supportive care to clients with smoking-related diseases are examples of tertiary prevention.
NP = Ev
CN = Ps/4
CL = An
SA = 2

25. **2, 3, 5.** Depression, psychomotor retardation and agitation, and unpleasant and vivid dreams are found in amphetamine withdrawal. Hypertension, overly suspicious and paranoid behavior, and touching and picking of the extremities and face are all clinical manifestations caused by the excessive use of amphetamines or stimulants.
NP = As
CN = Ps/4
CL = Ap
SA = 2

26. **1.** Skills that require providing smoking-cessation techniques, encouraging verbalization of feeling, and assessing for a drug dependency should be performed by a registered nurse. Unlicensed assistive personnel may assist a client to group therapy.
NP = Pl
CN = Sa/1
CL = An
SA = 8

SEXUAL AND GENDER IDENTITY DISORDERS - COMPREHENSIVE EXAM

1. During an interview with a client who has hypoactive sexual desire, it would be necessary for the nurse to assess which of the following?
   1. Hormonal imbalance
   2. History of sexual abuse
   3. History of substance abuse
   4. Absence of sexual fantasy

2. The nurse is collecting a history of a client with sexual aversion disorder. Which of the following findings should the nurse report as supporting the diagnosis?

    1. Lack of interest in sexual contact

    2. Anxiety over sexual contact

    3. Inability for close interpersonal relationships

    4. No marked distress or social impairment

3. The nurse is admitting a client with sexual pain disorder. Which of the following conclusions would be most important?

    1. The disorder is confined to females

    2. There is no real physiologic etiology

    3. The pain is not real

    4. The client can still experience desire

4. Which of the following should the nurse consider before developing a care plan for a client with sexual aversion disorder?

    1. The disorder is chronic

    2. The disorder is confined to males

    3. The etiology is fear and anxiety

    4. The disorder is characterized by an increase in sexual pleasure

5. The nurse implements which of the following nursing interventions for a client with orgasmic disorder?

    1. A complete physical exam

    2. Pharmacologic intervention

    3. Quiet and stable milieu

    4. Exercise regime

6. When planning care for a client with a sexual dysfunction, which of the following characteristics of the disorder is important for the nurse to consider?

    1. The sexual response cycle is always interrupted

    2. The disturbance is only in function and not in desire

    3. The disorder is only influenced by psychological factors

    4. The disorder creates significant distress

7. When teaching a client with sexual dysfunction, the nurse should emphasize which of the following points?

    1. Gender preference is key to the disorder

    2. Mutual respect is important

    3. Drugs do not affect sexual dysfunction

    4. Psychological sabotage does not affect the disorder

8. A client suspected of having gender identity disorder is admitted to the psychiatric unit and the nurse is asked to do a nursing assessment. What point must be the priority assessment before a diagnosis of gender identity disorder can be made? _____

9. A client with the diagnosis of gender identity disorder exhibits a number of clinical manifestations. What feeling must the client display before the diagnosis can be made? _____

10. The nurse identifies which of the following data as a priority to be present before the diagnosis of paraphilia can be made?

    1. Stress-induced fantasy

    2. Difficulty with physical intimacy

    3. Loss of libido

    4. Spontaneous remission

11. The nurse is caring for a client suspected of voyeurism. The nurse should assess this client for what priority clinical manifestation? _____

12. The nurse is assessing a client with the diagnosis of transvestism. Which of the following would support this diagnosis?

    1. The client has same-sex attraction

    2. The disorder developed early in life

    3. There is an inherent desire for sex change

    4. Substance abuse is often a comorbid condition

13. When treating a client with paraphilia, the treatment plan should include which of the following measures?

    1. Single-focused therapy

    2. Rigorous exercise regimen

    3. Short-term aversion therapy

    4. Long-term therapy

14. When interviewing the client with a suspected sexual addiction, which statement would the nurse find most indicative of the disorder?

    1. "I understand this behavior."

    2. "I need to be close to my partners after having sex."

    3. "I am okay without any sexual contact."

    4. "I have had many unsuccessful relationships."

15. The client with a sexual addiction has many treatment needs. Which of the following treatment needs should the nurse include in the plan of care for this client?

    1. Limited group therapy exposure

    2. Limited social contacts

3. Individual psychotherapy

4. Limited community involvement

16. One of the greatest risks for the client with a sexual addiction is the possibility of contracting a sexually transmitted disease. Which of the following interventions should the nurse include in the care plan?

    1. Adopt a disease-oriented treatment model

    2. Safe sex practices are necessary primarily for the promiscuous

    3. A physical exam is necessary if a sexually transmitted disease is suspected

    4. Treat the client holistically

17. Which of the following disorders is a priority for the nurse to control in a client with a sexual disorder?

    1. Influenza

    2. Schizophrenia

    3. Bipolar disorder

    4. Dysthymia

18. The nurse should question the use of which of the following drugs in the treatment of a client with sexual desire disorder?

    1. Antibiotics

    2. Analgesics

    3. Antidepressants

    4. Fungicides

19. Which of the following elements should the nurse consider before planning the discharge of a client with sexual dysfunction disorder?

    1. Power struggles can exacerbate the disorder

    2. Perceptual defenses are lacking

    3. Confrontation of old relationships is therapeutic

    4. The client needs to limit outside relationships

20. Which of the following is a priority for the nurse to include in the plan of care for a client suspected of a sexual disorder?

    1. Family history

    2. Psychological testing

    3. Drug therapy

    4. General history

21. The nurse counseling a client with hypoactive sexual desire disorder prioritizes which of the following nursing interventions?

1. The establishment of a working relationship
2. Referral to counseling for anxiety management
3. Referral to occupational counseling
4. Establishment of a drug management regime

22. When caring for the client with aversion disorder, which of the following is the treatment priority?
    1. Comorbid medical condition
    2. Interpersonal conflicts
    3. Anxiety
    4. The compulsion

23. A client with gender identity disorder is admitted to the hospital. The nurse who is developing a plan of care would plan for the client to receive which of the following?
    1. A drug for anxiety
    2. Strategies for coping
    3. Treatment to redirect the sexual preference
    4. Treatment for homosexual urges

24. When working with clients with high-risk sexual behaviors, which of the following is the priority for the nurse to include in the plan of care?
    1. Methods for promoting safe sex
    2. Consequences of risky sexual behavior
    3. Legal responsibility
    4. Treatment modalities for sexually transmitted disease

25. When working with the client with a sexual disorder, it is a priority that the nurse
    1. understands personal biases.
    2. gives unconditional support for client behaviors.
    3. protects the client from consequences.
    4. avoids establishing a relationship with the client.

26. The registered nurse is making clinical assignments on a unit that treats clients with sexual identity disorders. Which of the following should the nurse delegate to a licensed practical nurse?
    1. Develop a teaching plan for a client with voyeurism
    2. Instruct a client with sexual identity disorder on stress relief measures
    3. Assess a client suspected of gender identity disorder for clinical manifestations
    4. Document the behavior of a client with transvestism

ANSWERS AND RATIONALES

1. 4. Hypoactive sexual desire is characterized by the absence of sexual fantasy. A hormonal imbalance is only a theory and has not been proven to be an etiology. History of sexual abuse is not established as a contributing factor. Diagnostic criteria state that the clinical manifestations cannot be attributed to substance abuse or to a medical disorder.
   NP = As
   CN = Ps/4
   CL = An
   SA = 2

2. 2. Anxiety over sexual contact is the primary contributing factor to sexual aversion disorder. A lack of interest is not a sign because interest is not decreased. The client with sexual aversion disorder does not necessarily have difficulty with interpersonal relationship that are not of a sexual nature. Significant distress or social impairment are criteria for the diagnosis of sexual aversion disorder.
   NP = As
   CN = Ps/4
   CL = An
   SA = 2

3. 4. The client with sexual pain disorder does not lose the desire for sexual contact. The disorder occurs in both men and women. There maybe a physiologic component along with the psychological factors. The pain is real.
   NP = As
   CN = Ps/4
   CL = An
   SA = 2

4. 3. The etiology of sexual aversion disorder is fear and anxiety based. The disorder is not chronic but can be temporary. The disorder occurs in both males and females. There is characteristically a decrease in sexual pleasure for the client.
   NP = An
   CN = Ps/4
   CL = An
   SA = 2

5. 1. A complete physical exam is the best tool for diagnosing orgasmic disorder and developing a care plan. Pharmacologic intervention may or may not be indicated. Milieu should encourage socialization and interaction. Exercise is not specifically recommended for orgasmic disorder.

NP = Im
CN = Ps/4
CL = Ap
SA = 2

6. 4. A sexual dysfunction is a disorder that creates significant distress for the client. Whether the sexual response cycle is always interrupted depends on the particular disorder. The disturbance is in both function and desire. The disorder is influenced by physical factors, such as pain, as well as psychological factors.
NP = An
CN = Ps/4
CL = An
SA = 2

7. 2. Lack of mutual respect is the basis for many of the sexual dysfunction disorders. Gender preference does not play a role in sexual dysfunction. Drugs can precipitate sexual dysfunction. Psychological sabotage is a contributing factor to sexual dysfunction.
NP = An
CN = Ps/4
CL = An
SA = 2

8. The client is dissatisfied with one's role assignment. The client suspected of gender identity disorder feels dissatisfaction with role assignment early in the client's development. The client may or may not have anxiety over the disorder. The client's sexual preference does not factor into the identity disorder. These clients do not necessarily display an aversion to sex.
NP = As
CN = Ps/4
CL = Ap
SA = 2

9. Anxiety. A client with gender identity disorder will express anxiety about the disorder. Secondary sex characteristics and puberty provoke anxious feelings.
NP = Ev
CN = Ps/4
CL = An
SA = 2

10. 1. Stress created in a case of paraphilia induces fantasy. There may or may not be difficulty with physical intimacy. There is no loss of libido. There is no spontaneous remission because the disorder is chronic.

NP = As
CN = Ps/4
CL = An
SA = 2

11. **Compulsive need to peep.** Compulsive peeping is a diagnostic criterion for voyeurism. Other characteristics of clients of voyeurism include clients who are socially incompetent, heterosexual, and have few friends.
NP = As
CN = Sa/1
CL = An
SA = 2

12. 2. Transvestism is a disorder that develops early in life. The client is heterosexual and there is no desire for a sex change. Substance abuse is not a contributing factor.
NP = As
CN = Ps/4
CL = An
SA = 2

13. 4. Long-term therapy is indicated for the treatment of paraphilia. There are a number of therapeutic modalities that need to be employed, such as behavioral, interpersonal, and group. Exercise is not a contributing factor to the disorder, so an exercise regime would not be an appropriate therapy. Short-term aversion therapy is not appropriate.
NP = Pl
CN = Ps/4
CL = An
SA = 2

14. 4. A client with a sexual addiction has had many unsuccessful relationships. The behavior is a mystery to the client. The sexual encounters are fleeting and often with strangers. There is a compulsion for sexual contact.
NP = An
CN = Ps/4
CL = An
SA = 2

15. 3. Individual psychotherapy is recommended to treat sexual addiction. Group therapy is recommended. Social contacts are to be encouraged, and a supportive community is therapeutic.
NP = Pl
CN = Ps/4
CL = Ap
SA = 2

16. 4. A client with a sexual addiction is at risk of developing a sexually transmitted disease. Treating the client holistically is indicated. A disease-oriented treatment model is too narrow and does not meet the psychological needs of the client. Safe sex practices are for all clients. A physical exam is recommended whether a sexually transmitted disease is suspected or not.
NP = Pl
CN = Ps/4
CL = Ap
SA = 2

17. 1. Influenza or other medical disorders can contribute to sexual disorders that can affect performance. Schizophrenia, bipolar disorder, and dysthymia do not contribute to a sexual disorder.
NP =An
CN = Sa/1
CL = An
SA = 2

18. 3. The use of antidepressants can exacerbate sexual desire disorder. Antibiotics, analgesics, and fungicides do not affect sexual desire.
NP = An
CN = Ps/4
CL = An
SA = 2

19. 1. Power struggles contribute to sexual dysfunction. Perceptual defenses are acute. Confrontation of old relationships exacerbates the dysfunction. Clients need good support through outside relationships.
NP = Pl
CN = Ps/4
CL = An
SA = 2

20. 4. A thorough general history is the beginning of the adequate treatment plan for the client with a sexual disorder. A family history is important but not as vital as a good general history. Psychological testing is not the priority for assessment. Drug therapy is not a priority in the plan of care for a client with a sexual disorder.
NP = Pl
CN = Ps/4
CL = Ap
SA = 2

21. 1. The establishment of a therapeutic alliance and working relationship is fundamental in the treatment of hypoactive sexual desire disorder. Drug

therapy, referral to counseling for anxiety, and occupational counseling would be appropriate at a later point in therapy.
NP = Im
CN = Ph/4
CL = Ap
SA = 8

22. 3. The treatment of anxiety is the primary goal with aversion disorder. The existence of a comorbid medical condition would preclude a diagnosis of aversion disorder. The treatment of interpersonal conflicts would come later in the therapy. A compulsion is not a diagnostic criterion for aversion disorder.
NP = Pl
CN = Ps/4
CL = Ap
SA = 2

23. 2. Strategies for coping would be a primary goal in the nursing plan for a client with gender identity disorder. Drug therapy is not appropriate. Treatment to redirect sexual preference for homosexuality is not the treatment goal.
NP = Pl
CN = Ps/4
CL = Ap
SA = 2

24. 1. Methods for safe sex are always the priority in all sexual behavior. Consequences of risky sexual behavior, legal responsibility, and treatment for sexually transmitted disease may be included but are not a priority.
NP = Pl
CN = Ps/4
CL = Ap
SA = 2

25. 1. The nurse's personal biases will contribute to personal perceptions and thus the quality of care. Unconditional support is not warranted for harmful behavior. The client will learn from consequences and it is an essential part of therapy. Relationships are crucial to the progress of the client's therapy.
NP = Im
CN =Ps/4
CL = Ap
SA = 2

26. 4. A registered nurse should perform assignments that require skills that include developing, instructing, and assessing. A licensed practical nurse may document observed behavior by a client with transvestism.
NP = Pl
CN = Sa/1
CL = An
SA = 8

EATING DISORDERS – COMPREHENSIVE EXAM

1. The nurse documents the presence of a fine white hair over the arms and legs of a client with anorexia nervosa as _____.

2. A client is admitted to the hospital with a serum potassium of 2.6 mEq/L, a pulse of 48, and a blood pressure of 80/48. The client appears weak, complains of being cold, and is 50% below the desired body weight for the client's height. The nurse started an intravenous infusion as ordered. The client becomes hysterical, stating, "it will make me fat." Which of the following is the most appropriate response by the nurse?

    1. "Your physician ordered you to have this IV."

    2. "This IV does not have sugar in it, so it does not contain calories."

    3. "I understand how scary this must be for you."

    4. "There is no reason to get so upset."

3. The nurse is caring for a client with anorexia nervosa. Which of the following nursing diagnoses would be the priority?

    1. Imbalanced nutrition: less than body requirements

    2. Disturbed body image

    3. Powerlessness

    4. Risk for injury

4. After an initial interview with a client diagnosed as having binge eating disorder, the nurse determines which of the following to be present? Select all that apply:

    [ ] 1. A feeling of being relieved with the binge eating

    [ ] 2. Eating enormous amounts of food when in a restaurant

    [ ] 3. A history of laxative abuse

    [ ] 4. Eating when not being hungry

    [ ] 5. A feeling of not being able to stop eating

    [ ] 6. Continuous rapid eating of enormous amounts of food in a short period of time

5. The nurse should include which of the following interventions in the plan of care for a client with bulimia?
Select all that apply:

[   ] **1.** Encourage the client to avoid eating except at mealtime

[   ] **2.** Promote a weight gain of 3 to 5 pounds a week

[   ] **3.** Observe the client for 1 hour after meals

[   ] **4.** Encourage the client to identify foods that trigger a binge

[   ] **5.** Instruct the client to keep laxatives and diuretics in a locked area at home

[   ] **6.** Inform the client that there are no "forbidden foods"

6. The registered nurse is preparing to delegate clinical assignments on a eating disorder unit. Which of the following assignments should the nurse delegate to a licensed practical nurse?

1. Develop a teaching plan for a client with an eating disorder

2. Perform a physical assessment on a client with anorexia nervosa

3. Assess the family dynamics of a client with bulimia

4. Offer support to a client with anorexia nervosa who is tearful

7. The nurse should administer which of the following drugs to a client with anorexia nervosa to improve cooperation with treatment and decrease agitation?

1. Olanzapine (Zyprexa)

2. Fluoxetine (Prozac)

3. Amitriptyline (Elavil)

4. Doxepin (Sinequan)

8. The nurse is evaluating four clients with anorexia nervosa for admission to the hospital. Which of the following clients should the nurse consider for admission?

1. A client with a weight loss of 15% of body weight in over 6 months

2. A client with a serum potassium of 3.2 mEq/L

3. A client with a systolic blood pressure of 68 mm Hg

4. A client with a pulse of 55 beats per minute

9. The registered nurse on an eating disorder unit is preparing to delegate nursing tasks to team members. Which of the following nursing tasks would be an appropriate delegation?

1. Ask a licensed practical nurse to develop a class on eating disorders

2. Ask unlicensed assistive personnel to encourage the client with bulimia to verbalize personal feelings

3. Ask a licensed practical nurse to assess a client suspected of having anorexia nervosa

4. Ask unlicensed assistive personnel to take the vital signs of a client with anorexia nervosa

10. Which of the following nursing interventions should the nurse include in the plan of care for a client with anorexia nervosa who is hospitalized?

1. Encourage the client to talk about food during mealtime

2. Ask the client if any food, laxatives, or diuretics have been brought back to the hospital after a pass

3. Discourage the client from participating in nutritional counseling

4. Provide a highly structured mealtime with regular meals

11. Which of the following nursing interventions should the nurse include in the plan of care for a client with anorexia nervosa in the outpatient setting? Select all that apply:

[ ] 1. Set minimum weight limits in which the client may continue treatment in the outpatient setting

[ ] 2. Avoid discussing the client's irrational thoughts about food and weight with the client's family

[ ] 3. Encourage the client to be weighed daily at the same time of day

[ ] 4. Instruct the client to avoid preparing one's own meals

[ ] 5. Instruct the client to keep a food diary

[ ] 6. Assist the client with meal planning

12. The nurse should assess a client suspected of having bulimia for which of the following clinical manifestations? Select all that apply:

[ ] 1. Constipation

[ ] 2. A 20% loss of normal body weight

[ ] 3. Dental erosion

[ ] 4. Lanugo

[ ] 5. A serum potassium of 3.0 mEq/L

[ ] 6. Depression

13. The nurse is caring for a client with bulimia who admits to taking 120 laxatives and vomiting six times a day. What are two complications that are priorities and may be life threatening should the nurse assess the client for?

_____

14. During an admission assessment for a client with bulimia, which of the following questions is a priority for the nurse to ask?

1. "Do you ever become depressed?"

2. "What has your weight been doing?"

3. "How much do you binge?"

4. "Do you ever cut yourself?"

15. The nurse should assess for which of the following when evaluating a client with a binge eating disorder?Select all that apply:

[   ] 1. Compensatory behaviors

[   ] 2. Going to restaurants and eating enormous amounts of food

[   ] 3. Lack of feeling guilty about eating enormous amounts of food

[   ] 4. A feeling of not being able to stop eating

[   ] 5. A distressed feeling about the binge behavior

[   ] 6. A feeling of having no control about the eating

16. After evaluating the laboratory data on the following four clients with bulimia, the nurse prepares to admit which of the clients to the hospital?

1. A client with a serum magnesium of 1.5 mEq/L

2. A client with a serum potassium of 3.5 mEq/L

3. A client with a serum sodium of 138 mEq/L

4. A client with a serum calcium of 8.5 mg/dl

17. During a nutritional assessment of a client with a binge eating disorder, which of the following does the nurse evaluate as most significant in contributing to the binge eating?

1. A rigorous exercise plan

2. Periods of fasting

3. Weighing too frequently

4. Eating a diet low in carbohydrates

18. The family of a client with bulimia admits to the nurse that they notice their daughter gets depressed frequently. The family asks the nurse if there is an incidence of depression in eating disorders. Which of the following is the most appropriate response by the nurse?

1. "Is there a history of depression in your family?"

2. "Has your daughter been depressed over a certain situation?"

3. "Depression does tend to correlate with eating disorders."

4. "It is normal for everyone to have periods of depression."

19. The nurse suspects an eating disorder in which of the following clients?

1. A client who jogs 1 mile a day

2. A client who has a friend who is overweight

3. A client who has a history of sexual abuse

4. A client who eats a low-fat diet

20. A female client in the hospital with anorexia nervosa cries every time she has to be weighed. Which of the following interventions would be most appropriate?

1. Instruct the client to close her eyes when being weighed

2. Inform the client that she is thin

3. Inform the client that she needs to gain weight

4. Instruct the client to stand backward on the scale

ANSWERS AND RATIONALES

1. **lanugo.** Lanugo is a white fine hair normally present on the trunk, arms, and legs of an infant. It is a clinical manifestation that appears when a client is experiencing starvation and occurs in anorexia nervosa.
NP = Im
CN = Ps/4
CL = Ap
SA = 2

2. **3.** A client who has anorexia nervosa and is admitted to the hospital in an emaciated state is physiologically and metabolically unstable and not able to think clearly. The client is extremely preoccupied with body, size, and shape. The desire to achieve perfection is translated into weight loss. Telling the client who is very frightened that there is no need to be upset serves only to heighten the existing anxiety. Telling the client that the physician ordered the IV is not only scary, but also enhances the client's sense of having no control over one's life. Telling the client the IV has no sugar in it may not be accurate, because a dextrose solution rich in electrolytes is probably the IV of choice. It would be completely wrong to deceive the client. The best way to assure a frightened client is to simply acknowledge the client's feelings. There is nothing the nurse can do to make it better, so acknowledging the client's feelings is the most appropriate intervention.
NP = An
CN = Ps/4
CL = An
SA = 2

3. **1.** The priority nursing diagnosis for a client who is starving, as in anorexia nervosa, is Imbalanced nutrition: less than body requirements. Other

nursing diagnoses include Disturbed body image, Powerlessness, and Risk for injury.
NP = An
CN = Ps/4
CL = An
SA = 2

4. 4, 5, 6. A binge eating disorder (obesity) includes eating when not being hungry, a feeling of not being able to stop eating, and a continuous rapid eating of enormous amounts of food in a short period of time (generally 2 hours). The client also verbalizes feeling no control over the eating. The binge eating is a secretive behavior. With binge eating, there is no history of laxatives, diuretics, or purging.
NP = As
CN = Ps/4
CL = Ap
SA = 2

5. 3, 4, 6. Appropriate nursing interventions for a client with bulimia includes encouraging the client to identify foods that trigger a binge and to avoid keeping these foods, as well as laxatives, diuretics, and syrup of ipecac, at home. Having to go to buy these things makes it harder for the client to binge. A client with bulimia generally is slightly below normal weight or of normal weight and does not have a need to gain weight. It would be a client with anorexia nervosa who should gain 3 to 5 pounds a week. The client should eat when feeling hungry to avoid the temptation to binge. Fasting leads to binging. The client should be monitored for an hour after eating to avoid the likelihood of purging or taking laxatives or diuretics. The client should be informed that there are no "forbidden foods." Dispelling this myth promotes the healthy thinking that all foods are acceptable foods and that the key to weight maintenance is proportion.
NP = Pl
CN = Ps/4
CL = Ap
SA = 2

6. 4. Developing a plan of care, performing an assessment, and assessing a client's family dynamics are all skills that should be performed by a registered nurse. A licensed practical nurse may offer support to a client with anorexia nervosa who is tearful.
NP = Pl
CN = Sa/1
CL = An
SA = 8

7. 1. Olanzapine (Zyprexa) is an antipsychotic that improves cooperation with treatment and decreases agitation. Fluoxetine (Prozac) is a selective serotonin reuptake inhibitor used in the treatment of anorexia nervosa to improve weight gain. Amitriptyline (Elavil) and doxepin (Sinequan) are tricyclic antidepressants used in the treatment of depression.
NP = Im
CN = Ph/6
CL = An
SA = 5

8. 3. Criteria for admission to the hospital for a client with anorexia nervosa includes a weight loss of 30% of body weight in over 6 months, a serum potassium less than 3 mEq/L, a systolic blood pressure of less than 70 mm Hg, and a pulse less than 40 beats per minute.
NP = An
CN = Ps/4
CL = An
SA = 2

9. 4. It would be appropriate to delegate taking vital signs of a client with anorexia nervosa to unlicensed assistive personnel. Unlicensed assistive personnel should not encourage a client with bulimia to verbalize personal feelings. They are not trained to deal with what the client says. Developing a class on eating disorders and assessing a client suspected of having anorexia nervosa are both tasks that require the skills of a registered nurse.
NP = Pl
CN = Sa/1
CL = An
SA = 8

10. 4. Nursing interventions for a client with anorexia nervosa include providing a highly structured mealtime with regular meals. Nonfood related conversation should be encouraged during mealtime. A client's belongings should be inspected upon return to the hospital to prevent bringing in food, laxatives, or diuretics to the hospital. A client with anorexia nervosa would benefit from nutritional counseling.
NP = Pl
CN = Ps/4
CL = Ap
SA = 2

11. 1, ,5, 6. Nursing interventions for a client with anorexia nervosa in the outpatient setting include setting minimum weight limits in which the client may continue treatment in the outpatient setting. The client's irrational thoughts about food and weight should be discussed with the

client's family to enhance understanding and support by the family. The client should only be weighed twice a week. The client should be provided instruction on meal planning, including shopping for and preparing the food. The client should be instructed to keep a food diary and assisted with meal planning.

NP = Pl
CN = Ps/4
CL = Ap
SA = 2

12. 3, 5, 6. Clinical manifestations of bulimia include diarrhea from the abuse of laxatives. The client with bulimia is generally of normal or slightly low body weight. The client experiences dental erosion from the repeated vomiting. Hypokalemia and depression are also characteristic of bulimia. Lanugo is found in anorexia nervosa, not bulimia.

NP = As
CN = Ps/4
CL = Ap
SA = 2

13. Severe hypokalemia and dysrhythmias. A client who has bulimia and admits to taking 120 laxatives a day and vomiting six times a day is at great risk for severe hypokalemia and dysrhythmias that may be life threatening.

NP = As
CN = Sa/1
CL = An
SA = 2

14. 4. Although it may be appropriate to ask a client with bulimia if the client ever becomes depressed, it is a priority to ask the client if the client engages in any self-cutting behaviors. A client who self-cuts poses a risk to one's personal safety. It would also be appropriate to ask about the client's weight or how much the client has binged, but these are not the priority.

NP = As
CN = Ps/4
CL = An
SA = 2

15. 4, 5, 6. Clients with a binge eating disorder do not have compensatory behaviors such as using laxatives or diuretics or exercising. They eat enormous amounts of food in secret. There is a lack of control over the eating and a feeling of not being able to stop eating. Such clients experience a great sense of distress and guilt about their eating.

NP = As
CN = Ps/4

CL = An
SA = 2

16. 4. A client with bulimia who has a serum calcium of 8.5 mg/dl may need to be hospitalized. This client is at risk for tetany. Normal serum calcium is 9.0 to 10.5 mg/dl. Normal serum sodium is 136 to 145 mEq/L. Normal serum magnesium is 1.3 to 2.1 mEq/L. Normal serum potassium is 3.5 to 5.0 mEq/L.
NP = Im
CN = Ps/4
CL = An
SA = 2

17. 2. Periods of fasting or undereating tend to lead to binges for a client with a binge eating disorder.
NP = Ev
CN = Ps/4
CL = Ap
SA = 2

18. 3. Depression tends to run in families. There is also a 50 to 75% chance of an accompanying diagnosis of dysthymia, or major depressive episode, with an eating disorder.
NP = An
CN = Ps/4
CL = An
SA = 2

19. 3. There is a correlation between a client who has an eating disorder and a history of sexual abuse. An incidence of eating disorders does not specifically correlate with the client who jogs 1 mile a day, has a friend who is overweight, or eats a low-fat diet.
NP = An
CN = Ps/4
CL = An
SA = 2

20. 4. The most appropriate intervention for a client with anorexia nervosa who cries when being weighed is to suggest that the client stand backward on the scale. Simply telling the client to close her eyes may not be sufficient, because the client may not be able to control the impulse to look at the scale.
NP = Pl
CN = Ps/4
CL = Ap
SA = 2